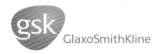

The expression "a picture is worth a thousand words" is particularly appropriate when it refers to medical photographs. Words alone can never create the profound impact of photographs that vividly illustrate diseases a physician might still encounter, as well as those that have already been brought under control.

Today, we no longer consider epidemics of the past as public threats. Yet, with ever-changing global dynamics, physicians must be prepared for the possible return of past scourges. An example is smallpox - shocking but possibly real because of today's new and frightening threats. President Bush recently announced that to protect Americans, the smallpox vaccine will be made available, beginning with the military and health care workers. But preparation begins in many ways, including an understanding and recognition of the physical, mental, and social impact these diseases once had on the population. Medical photography can help us reach that understanding.

GlaxoSmithKline, in its continual effort to serve the public welfare and the medical community, has commissioned an original educational series of four photographic books on the history of medicine from the Burns Archive of Medical Photographic History. These original works, titled "Respiratory Disease: A Photographic History 1845 to 1945," will encourage physicians to think about past medical practices and how medicine has progressed over its most critical century.

This collection, by renowned physician and historian Stanley B. Burns, dominates the field of early medical photography, containing more than 50,000 medically significant photographs. Many of them, complete with written explanations, have never been seen by the general medical profession.

Dr. Burns has published more than a dozen books and his collection has been the subject of numerous exhibitions. Recent presentations have been mounted at the Musee d'Orsay, Paris; Kulturbro 2002 Art Biennial, Brosarp, Sweden; The Center for The Study of the United States, Haifa, Israel; and the National Arts Club, New York. Dr. Burns' full collection of over 700,000 photographs are used by researchers, book publishers, media and film companies worldwide.

GSK is proud to sponsor this original Historical Medical Educational Series.

Chris Viehbacher

Chris Viehbacher
President, US Pharmaceuticals
GlaxoSmithKline

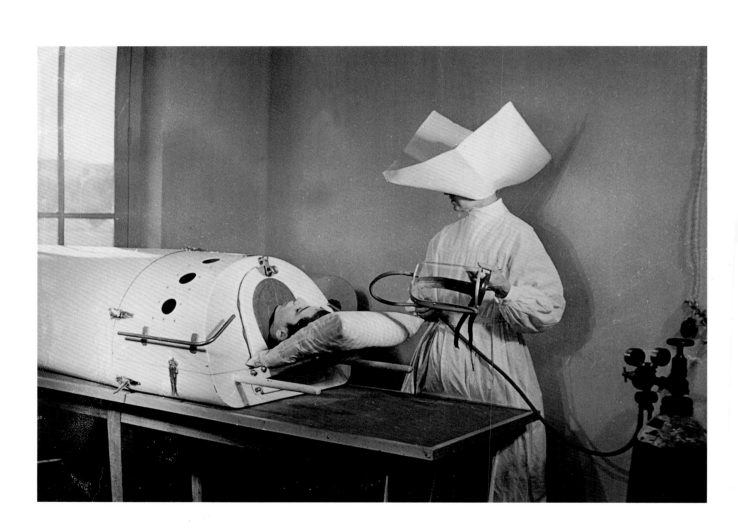

RESPIRATORY DISEASE:

A PHOTOGRAPHIC HISTORY
1921-1945 THE SEROLOGY ERA
SELECTIONS FROM *THE BURNS ARCHIVE*

STANLEY B. BURNS, M.D.

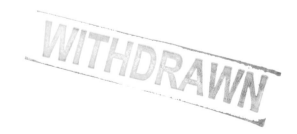

BURNS ARCHIVE PRESS

NEW YORK 2003

Colophon

This first edition of *Respiratory Disease: A Photographic History, 1921-1945 The Serology Era* is limited to 20,150 copies including a special cased edition of 1000 copies. The photographs are copyright Stanley B. Burns, MD & The Burns Archive. The design is copyright Elizabeth A. Burns & The Burns Archive. The text and contents of this volume are copyright Stanley B. Burns, MD, 2003. Printed and bound in China for The Burns Archive Press, NY, a division of Burns Archive Photographic Distributors, Ltd. NY. The book is printed on acid free 140 GMS Hi-Q Matte paper. The 4-color separations were scanned at 200 lines per square inch.

ISBN 0-9612958-7-2

Library of Congress Cataloging-in-Publication Data:
Burns, Stanley B.
Respiratory Disease: A Photographic History, 1921-1945 The Serology Era
  Includes bibliographical references: 1. Medical, History 2. Respiratory Disease
  3. Photography, History 4. World War II 5. Lung Disease 6. Infectious Disease
  7. Poliomyeltis 8. Stanley B. Burns, MD

The Burns Archive Press

Author & Publisher: Stanley B. Burns, MD
Editor: Sara Cleary-Burns
Production & Design: Elizabeth A. Burns

Photographic Captions

Front Cover: Invention of the Cold Air Oxygen Tent, 1931

In 1917, modern oxygen therapy was described by Scottish physiologist, John Scott Haldane (1860-1936). The cold air oxygen tent seen here advanced this therapy and provided a more effective apparatus for administration. At Philadelphia's Hahnemann Hospital, all of the first nine pneumonia patients treated were saved with this revolutionary device. One hundred twenty-five pounds of ice was placed in a special compartment to keep the air cold. In this photograph Dr. David Northrup is using the Barach Davidson Therapy Apparatus. By the 1940s oxygen tents had become a standard treatment for pneumonia and other respiratory conditions.

Frontispiece: Iron Lung with Oxygen Mask Apparatus, circa 1940

Two respiratory tract diseases arose with deadly virulence in the twentieth century, influenza and polio. Polio was a feared, deadly epidemic which lasted over 40 years. Death was usually assured when polio compromised the central nervous system centers paralyzing breathing and swallowing. The development of the iron lung to assist breathing was a major step toward saving lives and calming the public's fear. This photograph shows a typical iron lung of the early 1940s with a nun holding an oxygen mask.

Back Cover: The Respiratory Tract and Basal Metabolism, circa 1933

In the twentieth century, the means to measure basal metabolism was established by the measurement of oxygen consumption through the respiratory tract. It was found to vary in specific diseases, thyroid and body conditions. In this photograph, Dr. Francis Benedict, Director, Nutritional Laboratory, Carnegie Institute is measuring basal metabolism of a man at work. Benedict measured the basal metabolism of hundreds of men and women and evaluated with various disease states.

CONTENTS

PREFACE

THE SEROLOGY ERA

LIST OF PHOTOGRAPHS

    1 Patient in Respiratory Chamber

    2 Dick Test for Susceptibility to Scarlet Fever

    3 Survival of Large Through and Through Chest Wound

    4 Dr. Edward Trudeau and Camp Style Hospitals for Tuberculosis

    5 Lung Pressure Measurement in Artificial Pneumothorax

    6 The Drinker Iron Lung: First Successful Machine to Aid Respiration in Polio

    7 Endoscopy and the Development of Bronchoesophagoscopy

    8 World War I Poisonous Gas to Treat President Calvin Coolidge

    9 Heliotherapy and Fresh Air Treatment for Tuberculosis

    10 An Unfilled Promise of The Age of Serology: Tuberculin Antitoxin

    11 Postural Drainage in the Treatment of Tuberculosis

    12 Listening to the Lungs With the Ear to the Chest

    13 Positive and Negative Pressure Respiratory Therapies

    14 Emergency Iron Lung Ambulance

    15 Discovery of B.C.G. Vaccine for Tuberculosis

    16 Respiratory Testing and Treatment of Children at a French Institution

    17 'Artificial' Fever Therapy for Pneumonia

    18 Helium Therapy for Lung Disease

    19 Diphtheria Antitoxin Production

    20 "Germany Has 'Children's Hour'": Gas Warfare Preparations

    21 Baby Carriage with Gas Cover

    22 Post Op Ward Rounds: Changing the Dressing after Mastoid Surgery

    23 Modern Tonsillectomy, Photographed with a New Technique

    24 Wounded Marine in Oxygen Tent on Board Hospital Ship, USS Solace

    25 Penicillin Exposition: a New Age in Respiratory & Infectious Disease Therapy

BIBLIOGRAPHY

PHOTOGRAPHIC FORMATS

DEDICATION & ACKNOWLEDGEMENTS

PREFACE

As an ophthalmologist, a life-long collector and a historian, I am fascinated by our past and drawn to visualizing history. When I first started collecting medical photographs in 1975, I chose images based on both their importance as historic documents and as evidence of medicine's rich past. What I soon realized was their artistic strength.

In 1979, I created the Burns Archive, which is dedicated to preserving medical photographs and producing publications on the history of medical photography. By the mid-1980s, noted curators and artists became interested in medical photography as art. Marvin Heiferman curated "In the Picture of Health" in 1984, an exhibit of more than 140 photographs from the Archive. This was the first exhibition of medical photographs in a public art institution. In 1987, Joel-Peter Witkin edited *Masterpieces of Photography: Selections from the Burns Archive*. Since then, numerous major museums and galleries, recognizing the artistic value of these images, have started to collect and exhibit medical photography. These institutions now display vintage medical photographs of patients, procedures and practitioners to the general public.

What I have learned these past twenty-eight years is that art matters. Art elevates and stimulates us to see things differently. Art creates a different perspective and point of view. When medical photographs are presented to the public, the images are viewed and conceived in terms of personal mortality, human fragility and the vagaries of life. Terror and fascination draw the non-medical public into dialogue with these images. Although the art world's appreciation of vintage medical photography as art is laudable, my original goal as a historian was to present these photographs to my colleagues not as art, but as historic documents. I want my fellow physicians to visually experience the practice of medicine in the 19th century to help them gain a better understanding of the foundation of our therapies and patient treatment. As a physician, I am brought back to a different reality by these photographs. I see my patients; I see difficulties in therapy, I see personal challenges and I wonder whether what I am doing and what I believe in will one day be proven wrong.

GlaxoSmithKline has given me the opportunity to share with my colleagues these photographs on respiratory disease. This compilation is not meant to be an encyclopedic history of the topic, but to put the emphasis on artistic, medical photographs that will allow you to see the transition of medicine from yesterday to today. Many of the treatments depicted have long since become outmoded, but our predecessors believed they were offering the best therapy available. My hope is that you will look at these images as icons of our past and gain a better understanding of what we do and how we can better serve our patients.

Medicine's quest to unselfishly help and heal is one of mankind's highest goals. I am proud to be part of the medical profession and share these photographs to further that goal.

Stanley B. Burns, M.D., F.A.C.S.
New York, March 2003

THE SEROLOGY ERA 1921-1945

The 1921-1945 era contained the promise of miraculous therapies offered by blood serum components. Serologic study dominated immunological research. Unfortunately, for the most it part, it was a therapeutic dead end. Several photographs relating to studies in serology and vaccination are presented. This series ends with the discovery and mass production of the antibiotic penicillin. The course of respiratory tract disease was irrevocably altered in 1946 when the drug became generally available.

Respiratory disease remained the number one killer in this era. The development of the oxygen tent, fever therapy, heat therapy and vaccines allowed those stricken by pneumonia and tuberculosis to survive the acute stage of their disease. A new and deadly epidemic arose to challenge physicians, poliomyelitis. Various devices to treat the most serious complication, respiratory arrest caused by bulbar polio, are presented. The development of the iron lung, though saving many of those stricken, presented new moral challenges for the physician: making the treatment decision affecting who was to live and who was to die.

By the mid 1920s most surgical specialties had established national, fraternal and educational organizations. These groups raised the standard of care and defined who was a specialist. The result was increased confidence in the 'board certified' physician. Public confidence in these specialists whether surgeon or physician sub-specialist was reflected in photography. Posing and focus changed to document the importance of the procedure rather than the individual practitioner.

In this volume the treatment of pneumonia and tuberculosis are recorded and documented by therapies that seemed beneficial at the time but, in reality, offered no true cure. The threat of gas warfare was a concern in the late 1930s and opposing sides prepared their populations for this possibility. On the other hand, gas in various forms, chlorine, helium and nitrogen was used to treat respiratory tract disease. The oxygen tent with cold or heated air became an established treatment for pneumonias saving countless lives.

It is appropriate that this series end with a photograph of a common mold, *Penicillium*. Penicillin was the wonder drug that revolutionized medical care. Within two decades the common bacterial infections of the upper and lower respiratory tract that had dominated the practices of physicians and otorhinolaryngologists almost disappeared. Bacterial otitis media, mastoiditis, pharyngitis, tonsillitis, and pneumonias became relatively easy to cure. Asthma, sinusitis, emphysema, rhinitis and other respiratory tract diseases, related to allergies and environmental conditions, became the main focus of physicians.

The control of infectious disease has dramatically increased life expectancy. The mortality rate went from 40 years in 1845 to only 47 by 1900, but rose to over 75 years by 1980. Respiratory tract disease was no longer the greatest threat to life. Today, since we live longer, cardiovascular disease and cancer, which occur at an older age, are the leading causes of death. The photographs in this series attest to the long and difficult road patients and physicians have endured in dealing with respiratory tract disease.

1
Patient in Respiratory Chamber

Mt. Sinai Hospital
New York
circa 1924

The rise of America's leadership in medicine can be traced to the emergence of physiology as the central discipline of medical schools. The development of laboratory medicine in all fields created a professional scientifically based, medical practice that offered hope for conquest of all disease. Once it was demonstrated that almost all disease occurs because of some infinitesimal change in chemistry that results in physiologic alteration – it behooved scientists to discover the physiologic chain of events so corrective medications and specific actions could be developed. Whether the entity is arsenic, Vitamin D, tetanus toxin, cholera, AIDS virus or a single gene, each causes its effect by a specific alteration in physiologic function. In this photograph we see a patient in the respiratory laboratory at New York's Mt. Sinai Hospital. These physicians are studying respiratory gas changes. As a result of these pioneer experiments Mt. Sinai was able to develop one of the world's first hyperbaric chambers. The hyperbaric chamber allowed treatment of the bends in divers, permitted high oxygen concentrations/pressure for anaerobic/gas gangrene infections, carbon monoxide and other poisonings. The chamber offered a new and safer modality for the treatment of numerous other diseases. For proteinosis and other lung deposit diseases it is possible to isolate each lung alternately by intubation techniques then administer high oxygenation of one lung as the other lung is repeatedly washed with specially prepared fluids clearing the lung of residue. Patients with previously fatal disease are now surviving with these lavage treatments.

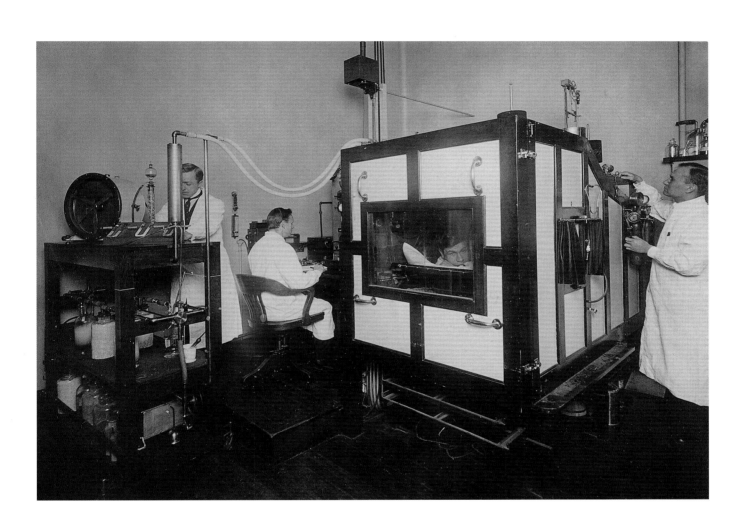

2
DICK TEST FOR SUSCEPTIBILITY TO SCARLET FEVER
NEW YORK
1924

Dr. Abraham Zingher, Assistant Director, of New York City's Department of Health, is seen here demonstrating on his own son the newly discovered 'Dick test' for susceptibility to scarlet fever. If a red spot appears after 24 hours, it indicates that the patient is susceptible to the disease. Within a few months an antitoxin would be available to protect the susceptible. In 1924, a husband and wife physician team solved the mystery of scarlet fever and provided therapy. George F. Dick, M.D. (1881-1967) and Gladys R. Dick. M.D. (1881-1963) discovered the cause of the disease, developed a skin test to determine individual susceptibility and then prepared an antitoxin for immunization. They published their results in various issues of the Vol. 82 of the *Journal of the American Medical Association*. At no other time in the history of medicine has one disease been identified and thoroughly managed in as short a time. The infective agent Group A hemolytic streptococcus, causes primarily a local infection of the throat. Symptoms include sore throat, fever, headache, and in two days a rash. Complications include anemia, meningitis, otitis media and rheumatic fever. In rare cases a septic and toxic form occurs affecting several organ systems. Death often occurred in these cases. Between 1820 and 1875, in the United States, scarlet fever occurred in epidemic form and was the leading cause of death of all the childhood infectious diseases. In the early twentieth century it remained a potent killer and the work of the doctors Dick seemed miraculous. The Dick test is the intradermal injection of a dilute infiltrate of a broth culture of a scarlatinal strain of streptococcus. If no red spot occurs it means the patient has a negative Dick test and has immunity to scarlet fever.

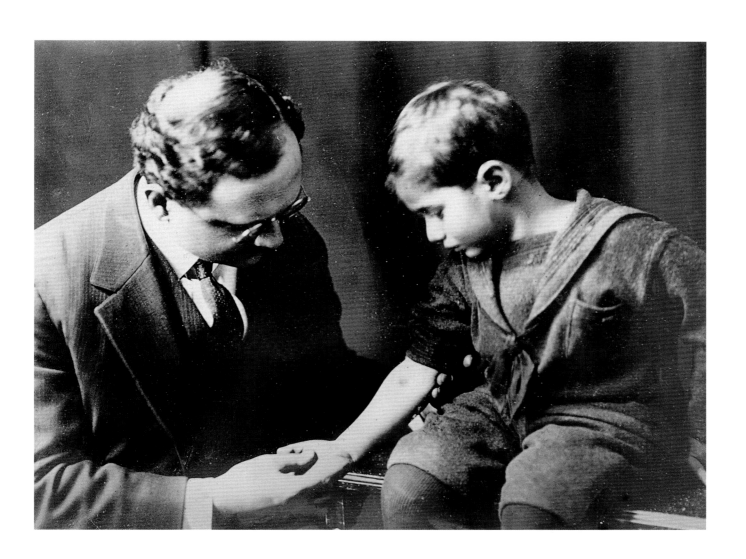

3
SURVIVAL OF LARGE THROUGH AND THROUGH CHEST WOUND
WALTER REED US ARMY HOSPITAL
WASHINGTON, DC
1923

Penetrating wounds of the chest were one of the more serious war wounds. Mortality was high even in WWI. The Civil War experience taught practitioners the life saving benefits of hermetic sealing. Antiseptic surgical techniques allowed development at the turn of the century of aggressive but safe lung healing procedures such as pneumothorax, lobectomy, chemical injection, and drainage. Development of Carrel-Dakin Solution in WWI thwarted infection. This soldier incurred a serious penetrating wound of the chest. After resultant infection and surgical procedures requiring removal of lung tissue, he is left with a massive chest and back defect and a healed fistula. The patient spent several years at Walter Reed US Army General Hospital in Washington, DC where this photograph was taken in 1923.

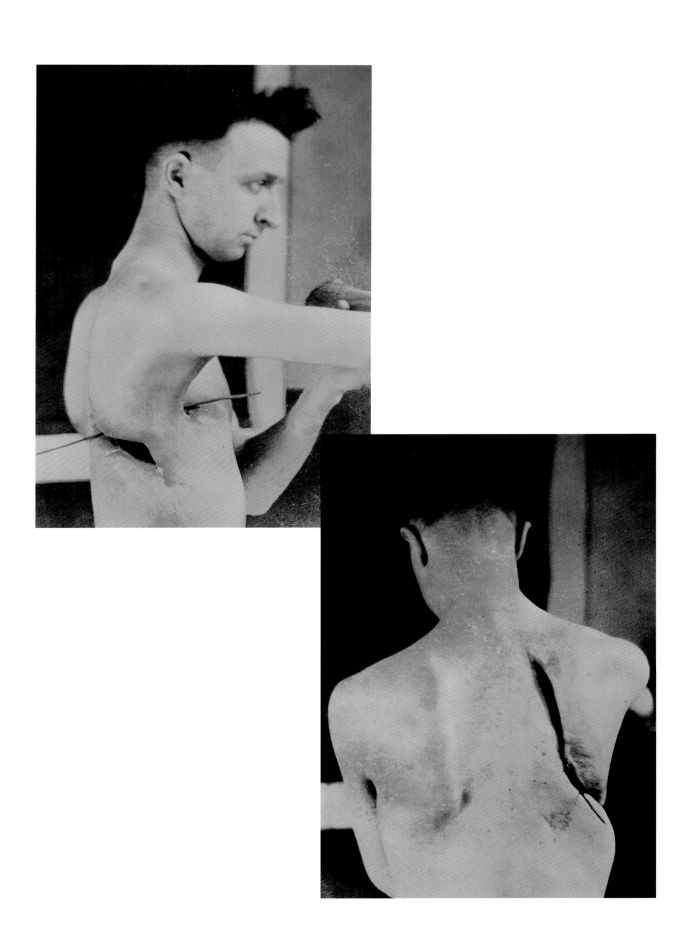

4
Dr. Edward Trudeau and Camp Style Hospitals for Tuberculosis
Colorado
circa 1922

In the last decades of the nineteenth century Edward Livingston Trudeau, M.D. (1848-1915) and others established the efficacy of rest and fresh air treatment for tuberculosis and other chronic lung conditions. By the end of the first decade of the twentieth century hundreds of outdoor hospitals, sanitariums and rest homes were established in the United States. The most common type of tuberculosis quarters were associated with an established hospital. On hospital grounds dozens of private isolation huts, as seen here, were built. Nurses and doctors made rounds on the patients as if they were on one huge ward. Many patients were housed for extended periods of times, sometimes for years. In the charity hospitals of the era, working class patients were housed in long wards with outdoor terraces or, in good weather beds or cots were brought outside for their use. In some localities public and socially conscious societies paid for patients to have some time of the year at special isolation camps. Dr. Trudeau's 'Cottage Sanitarium" and medical facilities in New York's Adirondack Mountains at Saranac Lake became a world center for investigation and treatment of tuberculosis. At the Saranac Laboratory, Dr. Trudeau had produced a tuberculin anti-toxin vaccine before Dr. Robert Koch, in 1882, announced his similar substance. Unfortunately, despite two of the world's expert's best efforts, neither vaccine offered much immunity nor help in ameliorating the disease. Dr. Trudeau's Saranac Lake facility remains an important institution in treating respiratory disease.

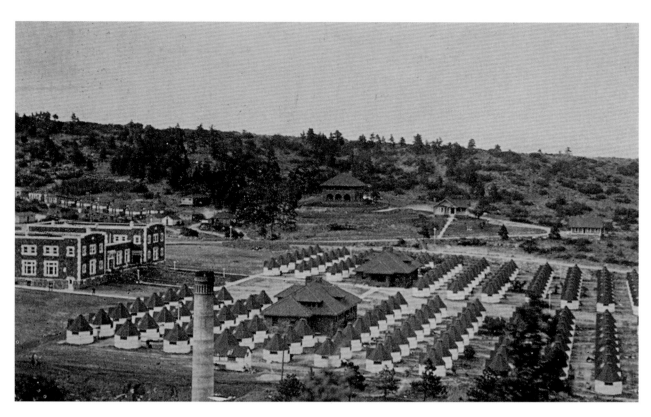

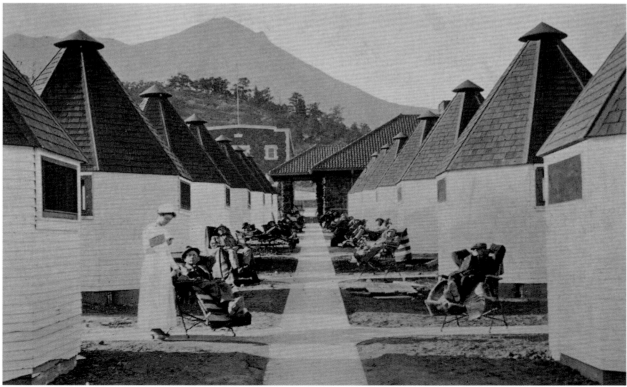

5
Lung Pressure Measurement in Artificial Pneumothorax
Germany
1932

By the second decade of the twentieth century, the treatment of lung disease frequently involved mechanical immobilization of lung tissue. This was accomplished by 'artificial pneumothorax', the insertion of inert gas (nitrogen) into the pleural cavity. The constant motion of the lung prevented healing. A collapsed lung allowed cicatrisation and encapsulation of tubercular foci. Pulmonary hemorrhage could also be tamponaded by the insertion of gas. Empyema and cavity formation from non-tubercular sources was also treated with pneumothorax.

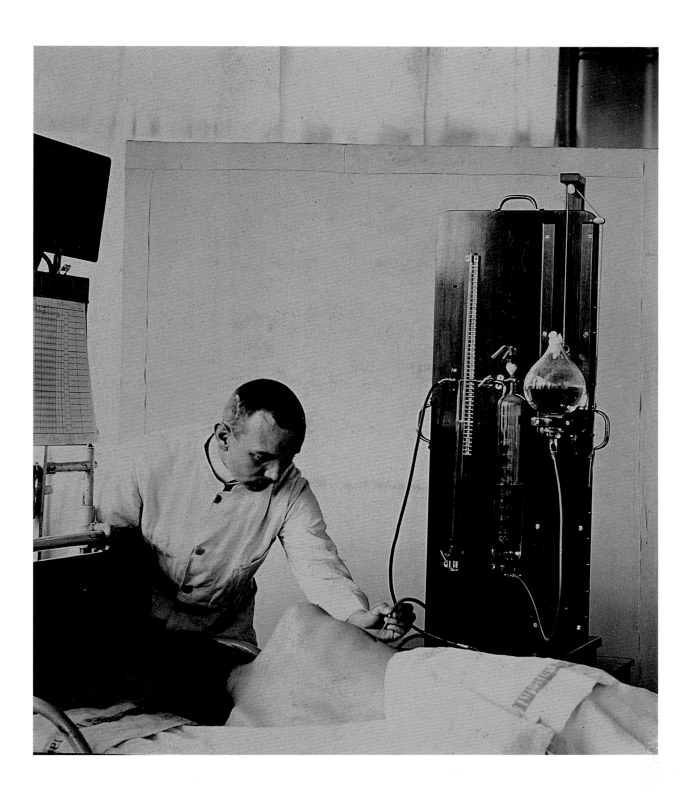

6
The Drinker Iron Lung:
The First Successful Machine to Aid Respiration in Polio
London
circa 1931

In 1928, Philip Drinker, an engineer at Harvard's School of Public Health, developed the first successful mechanical respirator, the Iron Lung, to aid respiration for polio victims. Originally Drinker developed a device to aid people accidentally gassed by leaky pipes, etc. New York's Con Edison Company funded the research in an effort to save lives and lawsuits. When Drinker saw children at Boston's Children's Hospital dying of suffocation due to respiratory muscle paralysis from polio, he recognized the 'blue face' and convinced physicians to try his machine. It worked. Then a moral question arose. 'Would the patient have to be machine dependent during their entire life until pneumonia killed them?' This was answered quickly as patients regained their ability to breathe independently. However, the time varied from months to years and, of course, some never recovered and spent their life in an iron lung.

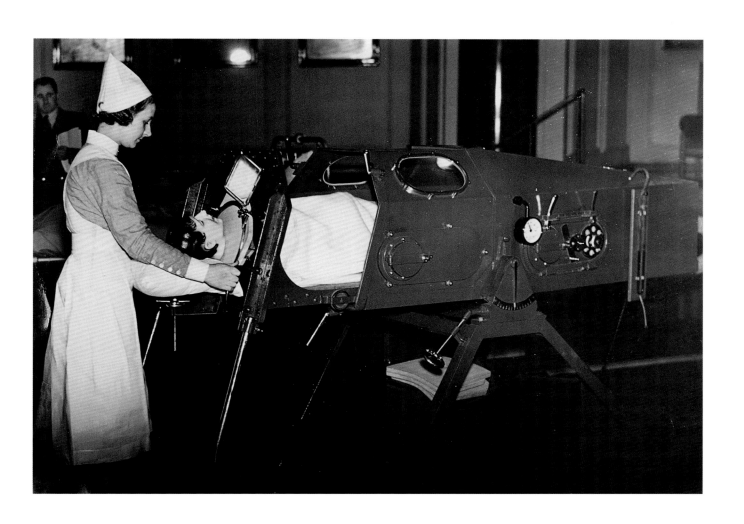

7
Endoscopy and the Development of Bronchoesophagoscopy
Dr. Chevalier Jackson at Work
Philadelphia
circa 1921

One of the greatest problems in diagnosis is the difficulty of observing either a diseased or a healthy organ. Physicians have been developing instruments to explore the interior of the human body since the early nineteenth century. The ophthalmoscope (1851), the laryngoscope (1854) and the otoscope (1860), advanced this knowledge in head and neck disease and created specialty fields. Dermatologists and ophthalmologists are fortunate to have their end organ totally visible but the lung and other internal organs are not as easily accessible. In this photograph, Philadelphia's Chevalier Jackson, M.D. (1865-1958) is seen performing a bronchoscopy. Dr. Jackson perfected this modern instrument and the procedure is associated with his seminal work. As with many medical advances, his accomplishments were built on the work of his predecessors.

Primitive endoscopes were developed in the first half of the nineteenth century for direct examination of the uterus, vagina, bladder and rectum. In 1853, Parisian urologist, Antonin Desmormeaux, M.D. (1815-1894), introduced a successful gas lamp apparatus to illuminate his urethroscope. His idea encouraged others to develop illuminating endoscopes. Dublin's F. Richard Cruise, M.D. in the late 1860s, developed a powerful light that allowed observation of the inside of the uterus. He then suggested that the respiratory tract and stomach could be similarly observed. A wide variety of medical instruments using illumination were invented and tested. In 1868, Adolf Kussmaul, M.D. (1822-1902), cleverly used a sword swallower in his unsuccessful attempt to pass an elongated urethroscope into the stomach while Louis Waldenburg, M.D., in the same year, designed an oesophogoscope with a laryngeal mirror attachment in the hopes of seeing down the tube. The designer of the modern cystoscope, Maximillian Nitze, M.D. (1848-1906), developed an electrically lit instrument and other improvements that were ultimately refined into a bronchoscope. In 1889, Victor von Hacker, MD (1853-1993), designed the first practical oesophagascope by lengthening and straightening the tube. Frieberg's Gustave Killian, M.D. (1860-1921), in 1897, adapted the oesophagoscope to perform a bronchoscopy and coined the term, broncoscopy. By 1905 several physicians were performing the procedure. However, it was Dr. Chevalier Jackson who modified the scope into its modern counterpart by placing a light in an auxiliary tube and creating a suction tube. This addition to the instrumentation allowed the main tube to be used for his newly created elongated instruments to manipulate and treat tissue. In 1907, Jackson published, *Tracheo-broncoscopy Esophagoscopy, and Gastroscopy*, the first textbook on endoscopy. He became the world's leading bronchoesophagoscopist. His clinic and school of endoscopy was the leading institution in the field. The field of endoscopy became a fertile ground for innovators trying to advance direct observation of internal organs from bone joints to heart valves. These concepts and procedures are now used in major surgical operations on the heart, blood vessels and sinuses. Miniature cameras, probes, snares and lasers are being sent deeper and deeper into the recesses of the human body. The reality of a minute miniature, robotic camera traveling the blood, lymph or other body system is not far in the future.

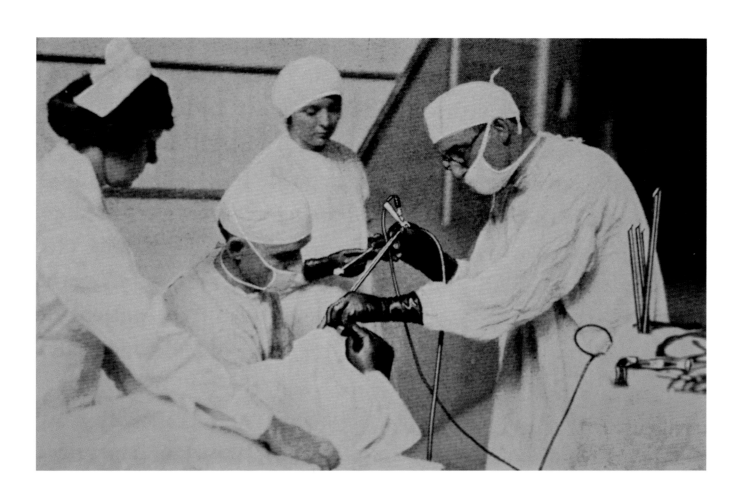

8
World War I Poisonous Gas to Treat President Calvin Coolidge
Washington, DC
1925

In this photograph, Lieutenant Colonel M.A. Delany, M.D. stands behind a cylinder of chlorine gas with the apparatus used to treat President Calvin Coolidge for a lung inflammation. Secretary of War, John W. Weeks, had been treated in this manner with good results and suggested the treatment might be beneficial for the President. Coolidge was said to have felt better after receiving the treatments.

In the pre-bacteriological age "bad air" was blamed for a multitude of diseases from malaria to tuberculosis. This theory was partially correct: tuberculosis and many other contagious diseases are airborne. In the eighteenth century when air's gaseous components were discovered, scientists investigated them as treatment. Until the advent of antibacterial agents, the administration of fresh air was a major therapy for several diseases. The entire course of medicine was altered in the late 1840s, with the discovery that nitrous oxide, ether, and chloroform could be used as general anesthetics. Scientists and physicians then experimented with inhalation of all known gaseous substances trying to find other magical properties. Because there were few regulations or restrictions on any substance, almost anyone could easily obtain any chemical agent from opium to cyanide. During the early nineteenth century, chlorine gas became a popular treatment for some lung conditions among "pulmonologists" or "phthisiologists," as lung specialists were known. It was not until World War I that the true nature of chlorine gas was brought to the attention of the general public. The Germans used this gas as a chemical warfare weapon in 1915 and killed almost an entire French regiment. Chlorine gas and death became intertwined in the public image. However, physicians reasoned that only large doses of the gas were deadly and for a time continued to administer regular doses to treat disease.

The deteriorating quality of the air in the world's cities has produced increases in asthma, emphysema and other respiratory ailments. Researchers must be supported in their continuing experimentation with gases for respiratory disease inhalation therapy, though this experimentation sometimes has deadly results. As the millennium (2001) started a volunteer inhaled hexamethonium gas during an asthma study and died. Although chlorine and hexamethonium, and other chemicals have been proven to be deadly, new substances will be created and tested for control and possible eradication of asthma and a host of other diseases. Research and experimentation, courage, hope and despair are all building blocks in medical progress.

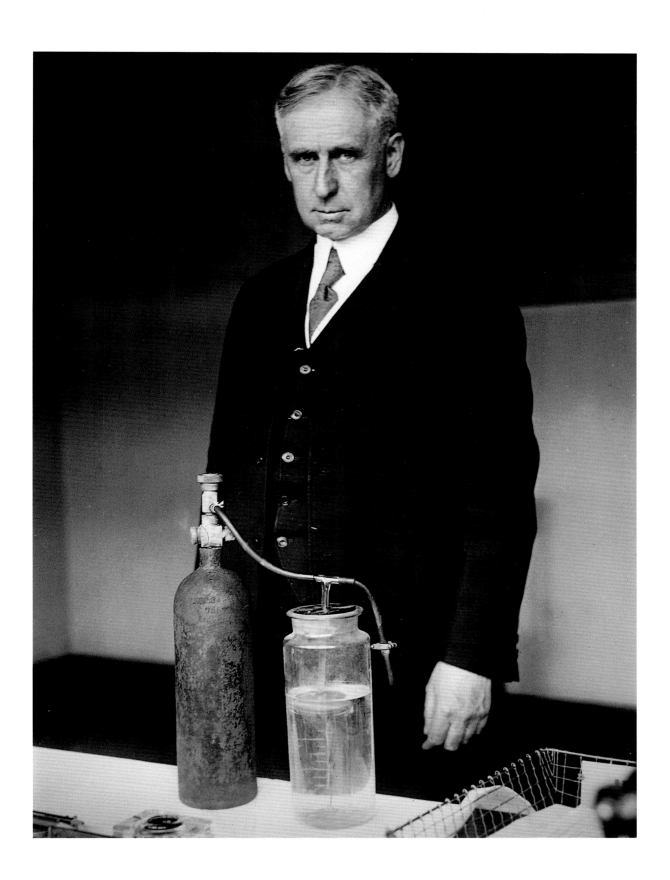

9
Heliotherapy and Fresh Air Treatment for Tuberculosis
New Mexico
circa 1925

By the 1920s, despite aggressive research, no successful tuberculin vaccine, anti-serum or chemotherapeutic agent had been developed. Most tuberculosis specialists recommended heliotherapy, exposure to the sun, rest and fresh air as the most beneficial, non-surgical, treatment. In the United States, Eastern and Western high altitude mountainous areas offering crisp fresh air and were thought ideal locations. This photograph was taken in a New Mexico tuberculosis sanitarium. Total nudity was preferred for heliotherapy. The warmer, western, dry desert states became the preferred destination for patients with asthma and other chronic lung conditions.

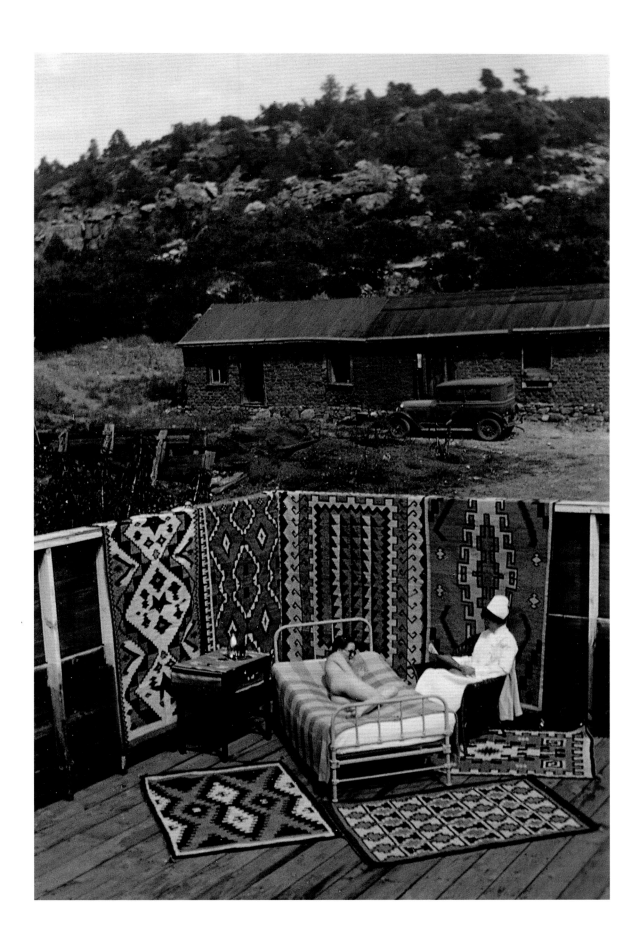

An Unfilled Promise of The Age of Serology: Tuberculin Antitoxin

Frederick Eberson, M.D.
University of California, San Francisco
1927

The remarkable immunologic findings and theories of Pasteur and Koch, in the 1880s, together with those of von Behring, Metchnikoff and Ehrlich, in the 1890s, set the stage for the study of immunology in the first half of the twentieth century. Two competing schools of scientists and ideology emerged: chemist versus biologist, and serum response versus cell mediated response. The direction of research was then influenced by two major discoveries: Dr. Emil von Behring's miraculous development of the first specific therapy, an anti-serum against diphtheria; and chemist Paul Ehrlich's development of the first chemotherapeutic agent, Salvarsen (606), for syphilis. The phagocytic and cell mediated studies of biologist Elie Metchnikoff had produced no therapy. Researchers became focused on the serum response to fight disease and create preventative therapies.

The first fifty years of immunology, in the twentieth century, was labeled the "Age of Serology" but it would prove to be a dead end. Only tetanus and diphtheria were effectively cured by the use of anti-serum. Thousands of researchers had developed anti-sera that, initially promising and helpful in a percentage of cases, did not result in miraculous cures. There were few diseases that didn't have anti-sera researchers. For lung disease, Koch and Trudeau developed an unsuccessful tuberculin anti-sera in the 1880s. Though some success was found in the treatment of lung disease with both Dr. Haffkine's anti-plague vaccine and Dr. Calumette's anti-tuberculin vaccine, they were based on attenuated organisms and not serum. Several of the serum based therapies actually prevented or ameliorated disease in some patients. This depended on the individual level of immunity, supporting the hope that a serum based substance could be induced or found.

In this photograph, Frederick Eberson, M.D., of the University of California Medical School, San Francisco, holds up a test tube with his new discovery "tuberculosis toxin". Dr. Eberson declared he had isolated "a filterable toxin produced by tubercul bacilli" and that "this toxin may lead to a discovery of an anti-toxin comparable to that used for the prevention of scarlet fever." He noted, "the existence of the toxin had been suspected but never definitely proved. Further experiments will be carried out in the attempt to develop a standardized serum which may put an end to the great 'White Plague.'" Unfortunately Dr. Eberson's therapeutic hopes never materialized. It was not until the discovery of streptomycin and other bactericidal antibiotic agents that tuberculosis would be controlled. A serum based vaccine was never developed. Tuberculosis remains a serious threat in undeveloped countries and to people with suppressed immune systems. A warning note has been sounded with the gradual resurgence of the disease in the general population.

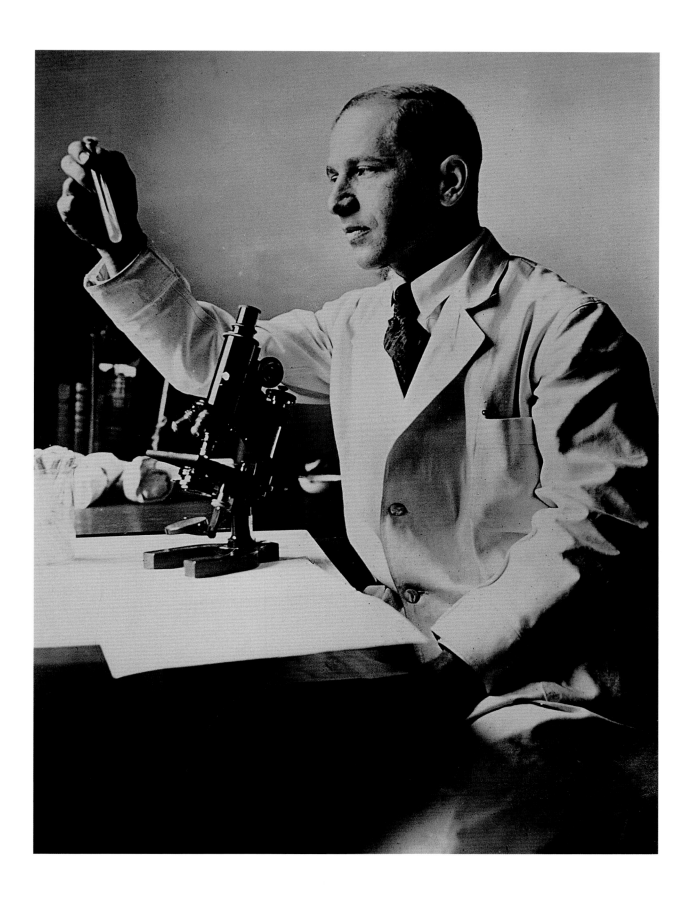

11
POSTURAL DRAINAGE IN THE TREATMENT OF TUBERCULOSIS
NEW MEXICO
CIRCA 1925

Pulmonary tuberculosis can cause progressive necrosis of lung tissue until an abscess, empyema or other adverse condition occurs. The abscess and other pockets contain accumulations of infective necrotic debris. When a patient changes position, especially lying down and turning, or bending over, the abscess will suddenly drain exudate into a bronchus. This will cause dyspnea and classic, paroxysmal, coughing fits. After a few minutes a cupful or more of fluid sputum is raised and the patient is relieved. This patient is being treated at a tuberculin facility specializing in rest, fresh air and heliotherapy. In addition to these conservative treatment methods, postural drainage for advanced pulmonary tuberculosis was a routine part of the therapy. Overhead bed pulley devices were part of the postural drainage regime. These pulleys supported a band which was placed around the chest of a recumbent patient, allowing the chest to be lifted upward, facilitating drainage. Stronger patients were treated with special racks as depicted here. This patient is hanging over a rack designed for postural drainage. This therapy was implemented several times a day with the patient coughing up infected sputum, ostensibly deposited in the sanitary basin supplied. Despite these treatments, if lung cavitation, empyema formation and deterioration progressed, the patient died.

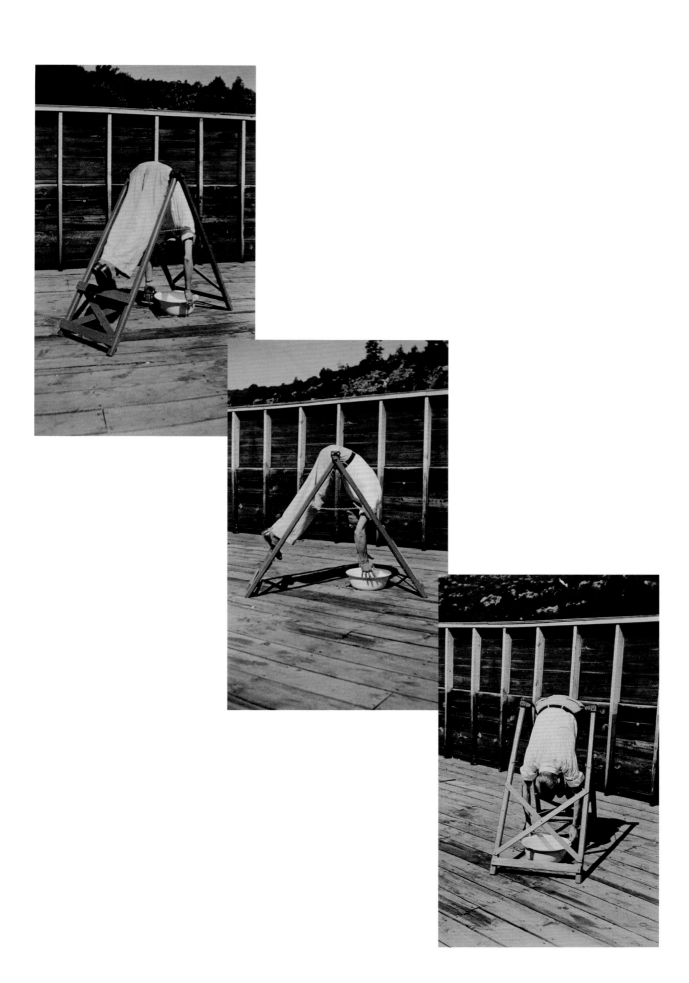

LISTENING TO THE LUNGS WITH THE EAR TO THE CHEST
FRANCE
CIRCA 1922

This photograph is part of a series of photographic post cards created to promote the facilities of a French post war hospital. Over 25 images are in the set. The photographs depict clinics, wards, laboratory facilities, operations, personnel and examinations. The photographs represent the documentation of the 'modern facility' and the medical image desired to be projected to the public. Photography allows better understanding of medical history as the pictures clearly show the times and practice methodology. Written words do not document position, status, and a myriad of other particulars that future historians may deem important. Most medical photographs have to be read with the understanding that medical photographs were almost always taken to show how modern and advanced facilities were, and how competent and up to date physicians were.

This photograph dramatically illustrates the difference between American and European medicine, medical practices and public image, in that era. There are no photographs extent of American physicians examining the chest with the ear from the 19th century and no twentieth century American physician would pose in the manner depicted. The binaural stethoscope - America's tool - was the symbol of American medicine, and chest physicians would never pose in a clinic or ward setting without the instrument. Diagnosis using an instrument of some type, whether x-ray or special internal or external examining device with laboratory confirmation, was the expected norm of twentieth century medicine. It's curious American medical photographs show that mystique while European photographs up to World War II do not necessarily show concern with instrumentation. Physician prominence was often the key and is vividly seen in photographs of the era. This status is a relic of the extremely hierarchal medical establishment that dominated European medicine for centuries. Perhaps the image represents closeness to the patient as a hand on a female breast and head to her chest may imply. It also may portray an era of physician arrogance whereby patient privacy and concerns are secondary to physician presence. Without an instrument it is only physician competence that you are relying upon.

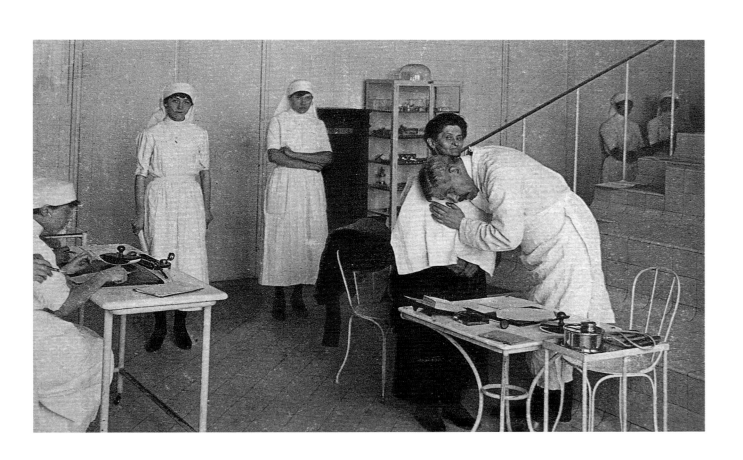

13
Positive and Negative Pressure Respiratory Therapies
Washington DC
1935

During the 1930s the introduction of Drinker's Iron Lung stimulated others to develop respiratory devices. The negative pressure iron lung of Drinker required a body size apparatus. Smaller upper body sized respiratory machines looked like medieval suits of armor and were nicknamed in Europe "curiass" respirators after the chest piece of body armor. They were less expensive and useful in emergencies because of their compact size. This photograph shows an adult wearing the chest respirator and a smaller, child size model is held by an assistant. Although this model has a complicated electric pump system, a less expensive, manual, negative pressure ventilation unit was available.

Although the iron lung was a miracle machine, its use forced many physicians into serious moral dilemmas during the epidemics of the 1930s. As there were never enough iron lungs available, children would be brought into a hospital and physicians had an intolerable decision to make: who would go into the iron lung and who would be left to die. Dying, blue faced children suffocating in their own secretions filled hospital wards and, to add to the nightmare, the physicians and nurses treating these, patients often contracted the disease. These children gave the polio epidemics their rightful, fearful place in the public mind. Few epidemics aroused such widespread panic. By the 1950s iron lungs were relatively plentiful. An epidemic in Copenhagen in 1952 resulted in the iron lung being eventually replaced by another method of treatment. A particularly virulent form of polio struck the city a year after the International Poliomyelitis Conference was held in the city. There were an exceptionally large number of cases with bulbar involvement. The epidemic struck 238 per 100,000 of population, a far greater number than any polio epidemic ever recorded. Many patients died for the lack of respirators, however, at one hospital, 27 of 31 patients treated in respirators died, raising doubts that more respirators would have helped lower the death rate. The hospital chief of staff was advised to turn to anesthesiologists for help. An anesthesiologist, Dr. Ibsen, recommended replacing the expensive iron lung respirators with the more available and simpler approach of manual positive pressure ventilation that could be accurately monitored. This was achieved by performing a tracheotomy, attaching tubes to a simple air filled bladder which had to be manually squeezed 24 hours a day. Medical and dental students working six-hour shifts for several months performed this labor to save the children. At the end of three months, the mortality of the iron lung patients was 80% and the hand ventilated patients 40%. Within a short period of time a mechanical positive-pressure pump respirator was on the market. Initially, the new procedure was not popular in the United States, as it involved a tracheotomy, and iron lungs were plentiful. Eventually the advantage of the tracheotomy and positive pressure pump became the standard therapy in bulbar poliomyelitis. The various models of the iron lung were relegated to medical museums.

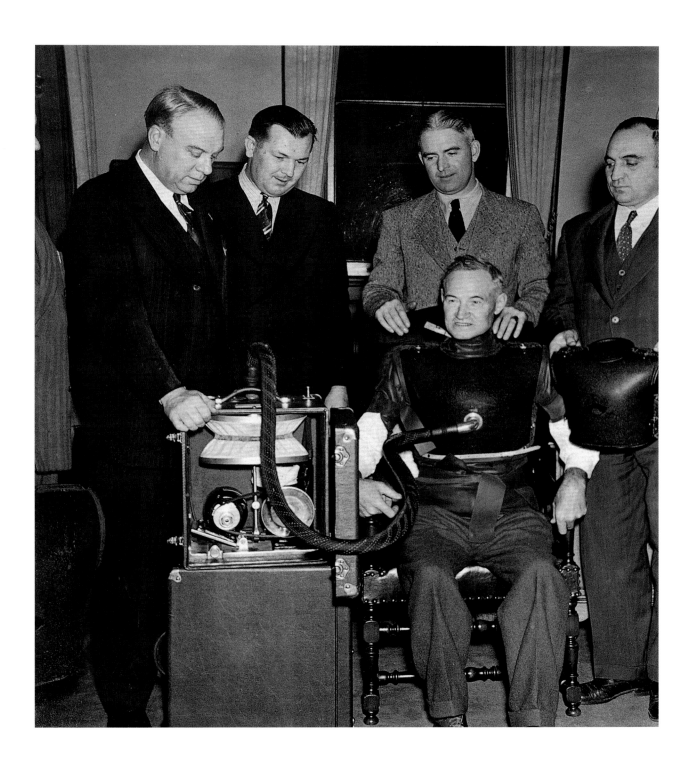

14
EMERGENCY IRON LUNG AMBULANCE
CIRCA 1937

Death from bulbar poliomyelitis was a frightening prospect for those infected, and total panic ensued as the patient realized he couldn't breathe or swallow. A good percentage of the victims died within three days even if placed in an iron lung. The prevailing philosophy was, perhaps, that the parents didn't act quickly enough when their child became ill and that if an iron lung ambulance could be developed it could save lives. The ambulance envisioned would offer early respiratory assistance and would avoid suffocation. The problem was complicated, however, as bulbar polio also paralyzed the throat muscles used for swallowing. As the secretions could not be controlled, aspiration pneumonia was a frequent cause of death of those in the respirators. The disease primarily attacked infants and young children but in the 1930s young adults also became targets. By the end of the decade, the disease, infantile poliomyelitis, was renamed simply poliomyelitis or "polio." When adults contracted the disease they were more helpless than children. Parents could carry their children to the hospital but ambulances were necessary for the adults. The creation of an iron lung ambulance had a great public relations effect as the fear of suffocation at home was somewhat abated.

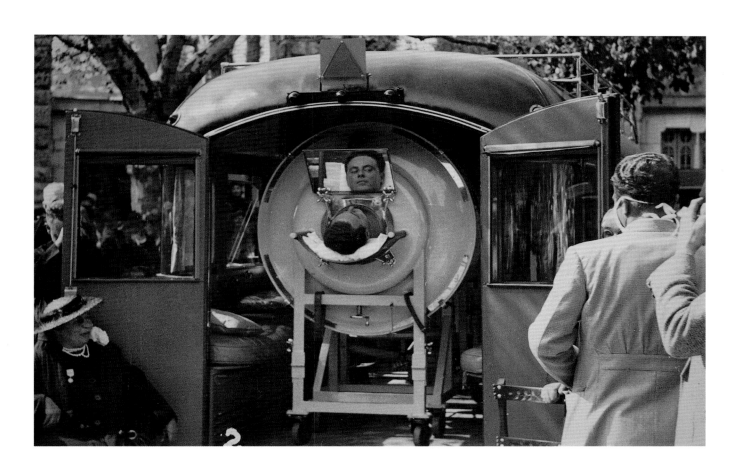

15
Discovery of B.C.G. Vaccine for Tuberculosis
Pastorien, Albert Calmette, M.D., Posing with his Microscope
Paris
circa 1928

In the first decades of the twentieth century, the development of vaccines and serum treatments offered cure and prevention of numerous dreaded diseases. Pasteur's bacteriologic discoveries and his development of the rabies vaccine resulted in international recognition. In 1888, The Pasteur Institute was founded, but it was not under his direction. Pasteur had suffered a stroke the previous year. Many of the directors of the institute over the next 40 years made landmark contributions to immunology. Their discoveries allowed the development of disease tests and treatment. These Pastorien's, as they were called, such as Emile Roux and Elie Metchnikov, went on to win Nobel Prizes. Effective tuberculosis therapy, however, eluded medical scientists. Tuberculosis was the number one killer in the nineteenth and early twentieth century. It was called "The Captain of All the Men of Death". Millions died from the scourge and tens of millions suffered severe deformity and chronic illness. Fresh air, sun treatments, surgical procedures, public health measures and slowing of the course of the disease resulted in a decline of cases. Attempts to find a chemotherapeutic agent, vaccine or serum treatment were only slightly successful. In 1906, Leon Charles Albert Calmette, MD (1863-1933), working with C. Guerin and B. Weill-Halle, produced a vacine that would ultimately be a major step in treatment of tuberculosis in the era before antibiotic therapy. Their B.C.G. vaccine was sub-cultured for 16 years and used as a prophylactic in children in 1921. In 1924, Dr. Calmette published his essay on immunization and control of tuberculosis. In 1927, after successful trials he published his definitive article, in the *Annals Institute Pasteur*, Vol 41, 'Sur la vaccination preventive des enfants nouveau-nes contre la tuberculose par le B.C.G.' Dr. Calmette, Director of a Pasteur Institute, is posing with his microscope at the height of his career.

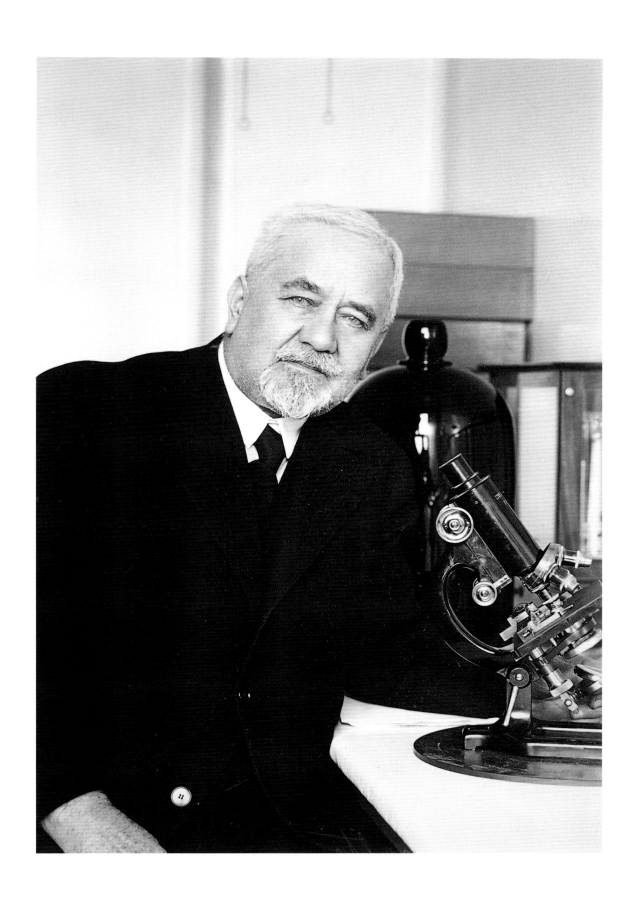

16
Respiratory Testing and Treatment of Children at a French Institution

'Surveillance de la croissiance: mensuration, gymnastique repiratoire'
'Centre d'Hygiene Maternalle et Infantile de la Nouvelle Etoile'
Paris
circa 1925

Respiratory tract disease was an important cause of childhood death and morbidity. Public health officials at the beginning of the century instigated preschool and school medical examinations. The school was often the place where working class children would have their first medical evaluation. Public health stations also evaluated the children. Childhood diseases quickly spread through grade schools as infected children came in contact with other children. Ascertaining who had been vaccinated and who had the common childhood diseases became important school public health policies. An important part of the physical exam in the 1920s and 30s was measurement of lung capacity. These children are having their lung capacity evaluated. Tuberculosis, pneumonia, asthma, and other respiratory diseases caused diminished lung capacity. Children with compromised respiratory tracts were more prone to develop infections. The evaluation of the level of exposure or activity of tuberculosis was an integral part of the exam. Skin tests and routine chest x-rays became part of the respiratory chest disease control program by the 1940s. This photograph was part of a series of postcards issued to show the public the inner workings of the children evaluation and vital statistic centers. Measurement of respiratory function was one of the most important parts of the exam.

Another similar looking device popular in French health circles was the medicated compressed air spray. The idea for a compressed air spray originated in French baths. In 1849, a Dr. Auphan adapted a water spray device to deliver medication. Dr. Sales-Giron invented a portable apparatus for water spray medication delivery. Bergson conceived the idea of breaking the stream of water into a spray by a blast of air or steam blown across its exit by a narrow tube. Laryngologists quickly adapted the device. Warm sprays were thought to be better but it was quickly discovered (in 1861) that no matter what the temperature of the water when it goes in the delivery tube, when it is nebulized, the resultant sprayed solution is approximately the same temperature. In 1866, Philadelphia's Jacob da Silva Solis-Cohen, M.D. (1838-1927), one of the founders of laryngology in America, introduced the spray device to American physicians. A spray device remains one of the important tools in treating all areas of the upper respiratory tract.

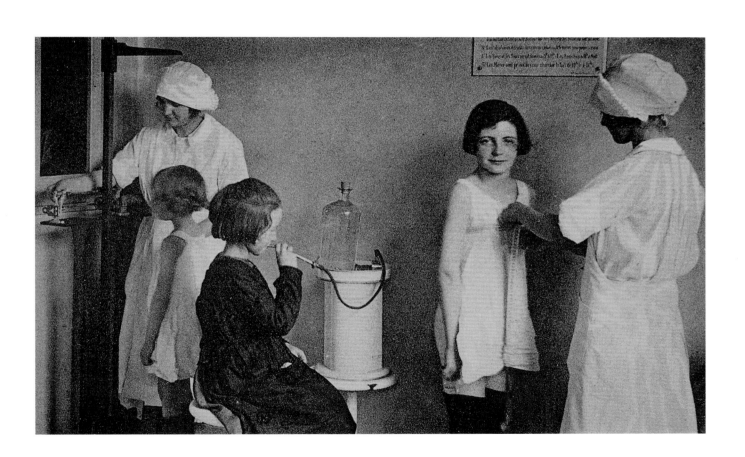

17
'ARTIFICIAL' FEVER THERAPY FOR PNEUMONIA
PITTSBURGH, PA
1937

Heating or chilling the body has been a part of medical therapy for centuries. In 1937, the University of Pittsburgh School of Medicine developed an artificial fever therapy machine for treating lung disease and upper respiratory tract infection. Similar in appearance to an iron lung, its function, however, was to raise the body temperature. It was also touted as a potential treatment for the common cold. Earlier twentieth century methods used the simple electric blanket appliances and steam. In this new device a metal cabinet encloses the patient to the neck; an electric fan provides cooling for the head; and a thermostat controls the temperature. Several of the devices were manufactured and installed in local Pittsburgh hospitals associated with the medical school.The fever device had therapeutic predecessors. In Native American medicine and hydrotherapy the sweat bath and steam room were important. These body-cleansing methods were actively used in treating respiratory disease. They had the added medium of warm air that assisted breathing. The warm air method was learned from hydrotherapy and resulted in a new medical apparatus for treating pneumonia, the hot air tent. Developed in the early twentieth century in the same style as the enclosed oxygen tent, it had the added feature of a long tube to deliver heated air from a boiler. The well-known feverous 'pneumonia crisis' with resolution of the infection once the fever subsided, stimulated the proposal to use an artificial fever as a therapy for lung disease. Some trace the modern concept for fever therapy out of a nineteenth century observation that a hospitalized, severely ill mental patient who developed a high fever in the course of an infection became mentally normal when the fever broke. Fever treatment research indicated fever was beneficial in diseases from influenza to rheumatic heart disease. Heating the body as therapy has been attempted in treatment of a variety of diseases from cancers to infections. When fever treatment didn't work for cancer in the late 1930s, an opposite view was taken and people were placed in ice.

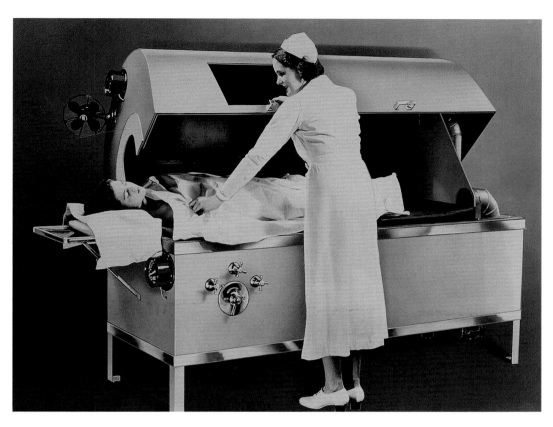

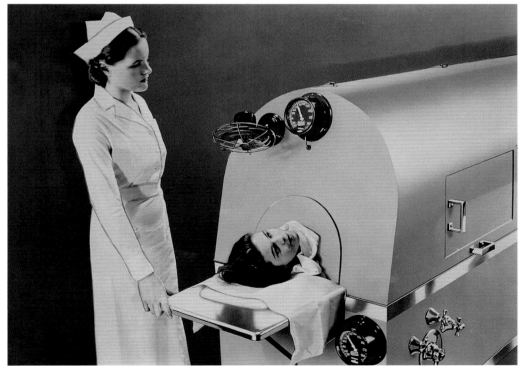

18
Helium Therapy for Lung Disease
Cleveland, OH
1938

In the endless search to find gaseous substances that could be used in treating lung disease, in 1938, helium was found to be beneficial. This photograph, taken at a Cleveland hospital, shows the apparatus used to administer the gas. Helium, an inert gas, was mixed with oxygen and found to be a more effective agent for 'artificial respiration' than pure oxygen.

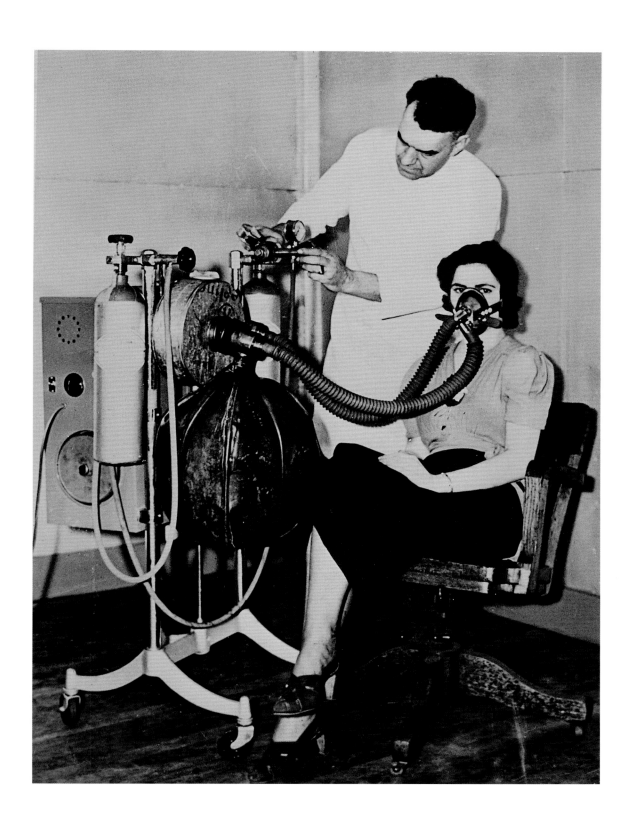

Diphtheria Antitoxin Production

Paris
circa 1938

Dr. Emil von Behring and Dr. Shibasaburo Kitasato discovered diphtheria antitoxin in 1890. It was the first specific therapy and turned the focus of the medical world toward the creation of serums to cure disease. This artistic photograph of large bottles of diphtheria anti-serum in the production stage was taken almost 50 years after its discovery. Few medical discoveries have received such continued attention. During the latter half of the twentieth century, diphtheria vaccine was combined with pertussis and tetanus in a combination injection, the noted 'DPT' series. In December 2002 the vaccine was further improved. Now for the first time Hepatitis B and polio are included with the DPT combination and infants are protected against five diseases. The vaccine, Pediarix, must be given three times at 2, 4 and 6 months of age. The advantage is that instead of 15 injections during the first year of life only 9 injections are needed. Many parents, and their babies, object to the multiple injections.

There is a segment of the population that can best be described as 'anti-vaccination'. These individuals have not considered that the major advance of medicine has been in preventive therapies. History shows vaccination, especially those against viral diseases, is the only effective remedy. While miracle antibiotics can treat diphtheria and other susceptible bacterial diseases, it is far better to not contract the disease. Only vaccination allows that. The images of the severe complications of these childhood diseases seen in this series attest to the advance of medicine and the miracle of vaccination. This particular photograph comes from a series of images documenting the manufacture of the anti-serum. It was taken in the popular European Bauhaus photographic style that, among other things, reflected a modernist concern and fascination with industrial production. Among the most interesting medical manufacturing processes was diphtheria antitoxin production. These images were created to project an aura of abundance, uniformity and order by documenting rows of materials. The composition was to represent the beauty of the modern age. This 'new photography' was most popular in Germany but had many followers around the world. Photographs of medical subjects can be dated fairly accurately because physicians in their advertising and documentation imagery usually attempted to be portrayed in the most modern of styles.

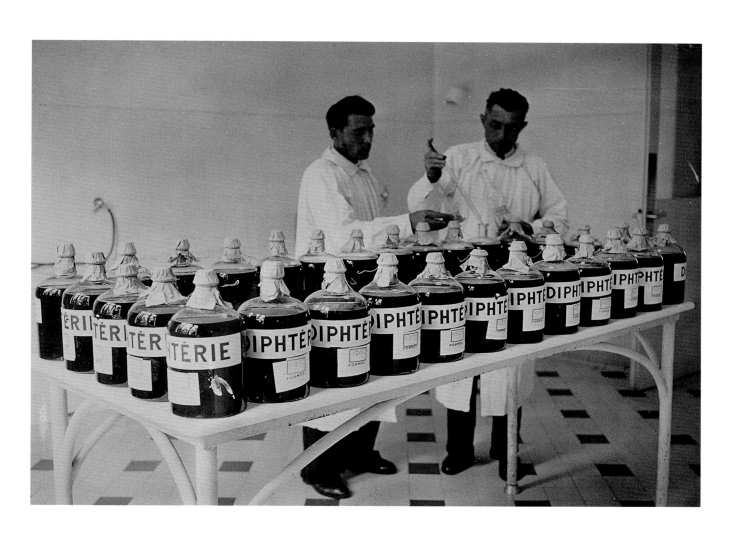

20
"Germany Has 'Children's Hour'": Gas Warfare Preparations
Berlin
1938

The fear of gas warfare prior to World War II had both the Allied and Axis nations preparing for the 'inevitable.' In 1938, when Adolf Hitler pushed east and demanded partial annexation of Czechoslovakia he was concerned that the drive might backfire and Berlin would be attacked. To prepare the city, he had school children don gas masks and undergo gas attack drills. In order to make the drills more realistic the children were required to pass through a gas filled chamber wearing their masks. Gas warfare never materialized in World War II. Only one major violation occurred before World War II, when Italy used mustard gas against the Ethiopians in the Abyssinia campaign in 1936. While gas was not used in the war, researchers continued to develop toxic agents. Germany created the most potent agent-nerve gas. These odorless, tasteless gases were far more powerful than the phosogene or mustard gases of World War I. Tabun, sarin, and soman, similar in chemical composition to insecticides, were gases that killed within minutes. Although the Germans manufactured over 12,000 tons of tabun it was never used. The Allies had no comparable gas agent and had no knowledge of the nerve gases until the war ended, which made the rumor of Hitler's new and secret, powerful weapon a reality. At the end of World War II over 1000 tons of tabun and sarin were removed from German depositories and sent to the United States. The total amount of gas manufactured by the Nazis was substantial. At one storage facility in St. Georgian in Austria, 250,000 tons of various nerve and conventional gas were found in storage dumps. Germany did manage to use large amounts of poison gas in World War II, but not against combatants. About 5 million of the 6 million Jews murdered in the war were killed by Zyklon B, a cyanide based gas. Prior to the development of the efficient gas chambers at Treblinka, Sobibor, Chelmno and Auschwitz, carbon monoxide gas was used. It was an inefficient system, as the carbon monoxide was created by gasoline powered trucks with the victims locked inside. In the 1980s Iraqi dictator Saddham Hussein used mustard gas against Kurd civilians. Perhaps the poison gas lesson of the twentieth century is that rogue nations prefer to use poison gas against helpless civilians rather than risk retaliation by another nation. As shown in World War I, an opposing belligerent nation will develop and use its own and better gas against the initial attackers and also develop protective gear. The first gas attack (using chlorine) by the Germans against the French at Ypres on April 22, 1915, was devastating: five thousand died, over 10,000 were wounded and the front collapsed. Luckily, the Germans did not take advantage of the situation. On May 1st, just 9 days later, a German infantry attack preceded by a chlorine gas attack was stopped, as the Allies had shipped gas masks to the front lines. Most poison gases required respiratory inspiration to be effective. Some of the newer gases can now enter the body through the skin, which requires the use of protective clothing as well as gas masks. Hence, gas masks, as well as protective clothing, are necessary for full protection.

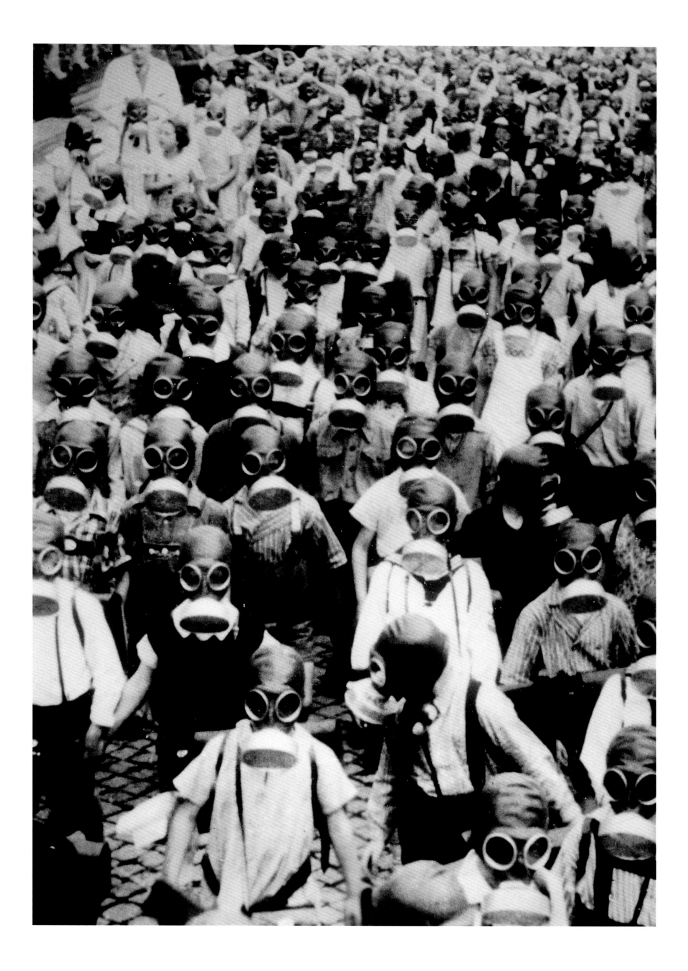

21
Baby Carriage with Gas Cover
England
1938

England in the late 1930s was preparing for war with Germany. Since Germany initiated gas warfare in World War I, and again, seemed to be preparing for gas warfare, the prevailing consensus in England was that gas warfare was a distinct probability. At the time of the 'Munich Crisis' over Germany's occupation of Czechoslovakia's Sudetenland, in September of 1938, the British Ministry of Home Security distributed 38,000,000 gas masks to its citizens. As part of the goal to offer its citizens comprehensive gas protection and to make the population feel protected, English researchers developed almost every conceivable device to protect against a gas attack. Every home had gas masks. To allay mothers' fears, baby gas outfits were available. No protective device seemed more outrageous than this special baby carriage outfitted with a protective hood and gas respirator. A mother wearing her mask could supposedly take her infant out for a walk without fear. England spent a major portion of its home defense expenditures on gas war preparation - to the detriment of building adequate antiaircraft defenses. When war came it was in the form of Luftwaffe bombers and V2 rockets. London and other cities were almost helpless under the constant air raids. Concern about an across-the-channel invasion could never be carried out as the Germans couldn't make or command enough vessels to bring an Army across. Also, the English had a rugged coastline, much of it flanked by imposing cliffs, so there were few easy landing areas. The English informed the Germans about their intended use of "Greek Fire". England, who controlled much of the world's oil, had laid pipes out into the water and demonstrated to the Germans how quickly oil could be run through them and set their troops on fire. An attacking army would have been burned before they reached the beaches.

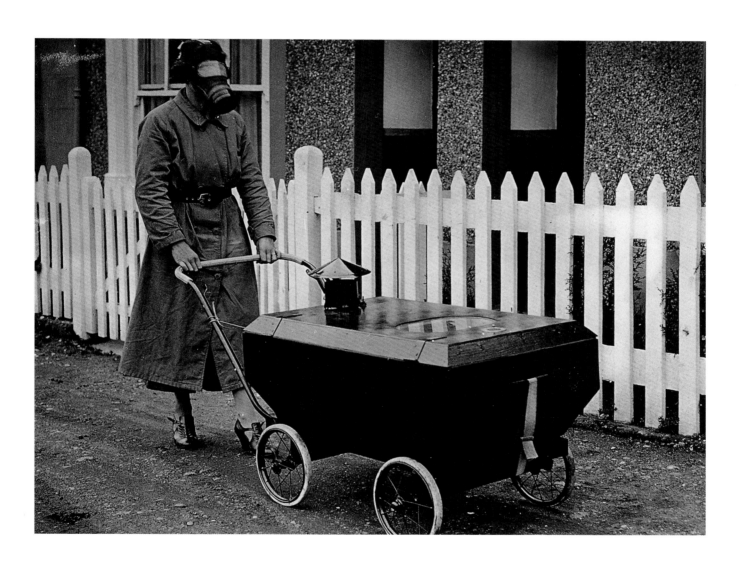

Post Op Ward Rounds, Changing the Dressing after Mastoid Surgery

CIRCA 1930

These physicians and nurses are changing the dressing and packing the mastoid area. Abscess cavities were packed with dressings soaked in antiseptics. A dressing cart by the nurse on the left contains unfurled bandages and medications. In pre-antibiotic days otitis media often extended into the mastoid air cells and resulted in a chronic mastoiditis. At times abscesses developed requiring emergency surgery, as extension into the brain resulted in death. To prevent these abscesses chronic mastoiditis was frequently operated upon. It became one of the most frequently performed procedures. Though it often resulted in loss of hearing. One of the advancements in the twentieth century was the development of procedures that saved hearing. In the surgical treatment of chronic suppurative otitis media it was recognized that multiple approaches were necessary. The disease could be removed through the ear canal or via a mastoid approach combined with tympanoplasty. Two basic mastoidectomy procedures evolved in the mid-twentieth century; the 'canal wall down' and 'the canal wall up' techniques. The canal wall down procedure, a modification of the mastoidectomy, described by Gustave Bondy, M.D. in 1910, became for most surgeons the procedure of choice. To obliterate large cavities various techniques were eventually developed, from muscle flap insertions to bone grafts. The advent of antibiotics changed the management of otitis media and mastoiditis. The night emergency cortical mastoidectomy procedure became relegated to history.

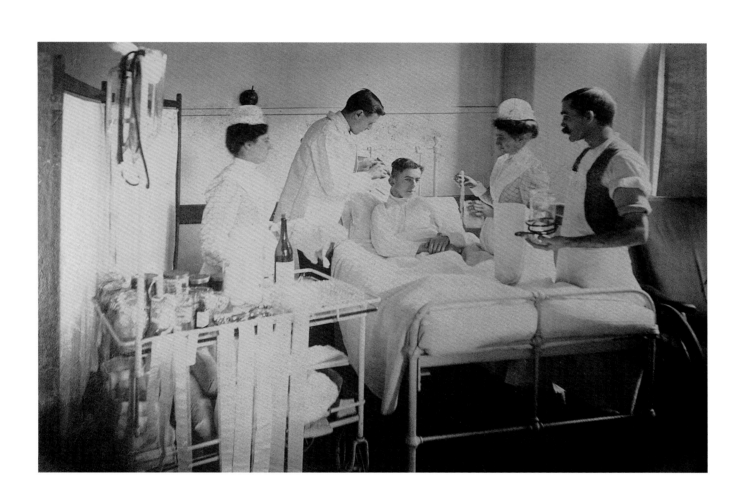

Modern Tonsillectomy, Photographed with a New Technique

1940

At the end of the 1930s, a new dramatic lighting style of professional, operative photography became established. In these photographs a spot light highlight the procedure while the physicians remain shadowed. The emphasis was on the patient and technique and not the surgeon, symbolizing a change in ideology. In the early twentieth century the 'master surgeon photograph' prevailed. It was an era of surgical specialty development. There were few innovators, and they were important. The surgical clinics they established became meccas of learning, the names legend: Halstead, Mayo, Cushing, Ochsner, Kelly, Crile, etc. The Hopkins residency system taken up by American institutions produced, by 1940, two new generations of competent physicians. They were providing modern techniques to the public. Specialty organizations provided credentials and the atmosphere was one of surgical competence. It was no longer necessary to have the one master surgeon, the innovator, to operate on you. Good surgery was available to the general public. This was one of the major achievements of medicine in the first half of the century.

The surgeons in this photograph are performing a tonsillectomy, one of the most common upper respiratory tract operations and one of the oldest developed throat operations. By the late 1940s simple tonsillectomies and adenoidectomies were being performed by general practitioners in their offices. The author can attest to this as he had his tonsils removed under ether anesthesia by his GP in the office in 1944.

A written description of tonsillectomy was recorded by Aetius of Amida in the early sixth century; "in tonsillectomy the tonsil is pulled forward by a hook, and the projecting part cut off by a knife; care should be taken to include the prominent portion, as there is danger of hemorrhage if the gland is excised too deeply." The serious complication of hemorrhage was recognized early, and by the Middle Ages cautery was used in the procedure. By the Renaissance tonsillar abscesses were routinely drained, and if they couldn't be drained, the tonsils were removed. By the seventeenth century ligatures were used to tie the base of the tonsils before excising. Benjamin Bell, M.D. (1749-1806) devised a uvulotome and a double snare for ligation of the tonsils. The basic uvulotome was developed in Norway in the sixteenth century to treat a peculiar infection of the throat that lead to such swelling of the fauces and uvula that the patient would suffocate. A peasant, Canute of Thornbern, developed an instrument that could cut off the uvula with great speed. By the eighteenth century the ligature technique was favored by many physicians who simply tightened the ligature around the base of the tonsil for a day or two until the tonsil fell off. Pierre-Joseph Desault, M.D. (1744-1795) modified a cystotome into a tonsillotome type instrument that amputated the tonsil.

The modern tonsillotome snare was developed in 1828, by Philip Sang Physick, M.D. (1768-1837) of Philadelphia. He was disgusted with the grueling, twelve-hour procedure of tonsil strangulation with a wire that was popular in the early nineteenth century. In 1828, he redesigned Bell's uvulotome to hold the tissues better and to make a larger and cleaner cut. It was the first modern guillotine technique tonsillotome. Morrell Mackensie, M.D. (1837-1892) provided some important general refinements, including a reversible handle so a surgeon could remove both tonsils easily and a double tonsillotome to remove both tonsils at once. In the twentieth century numerous modifications were made reducing hemorrhage, and operating time. Safer operating position, a gag to catch blood and brief chloroform anesthesia allowed the procedure to be easily done. Today indications for tonsillectomy and adenoidectomy remain controversial. The operation, once the most popular of throat procedures, is now elective and the benefits considered in the total care of the patient.

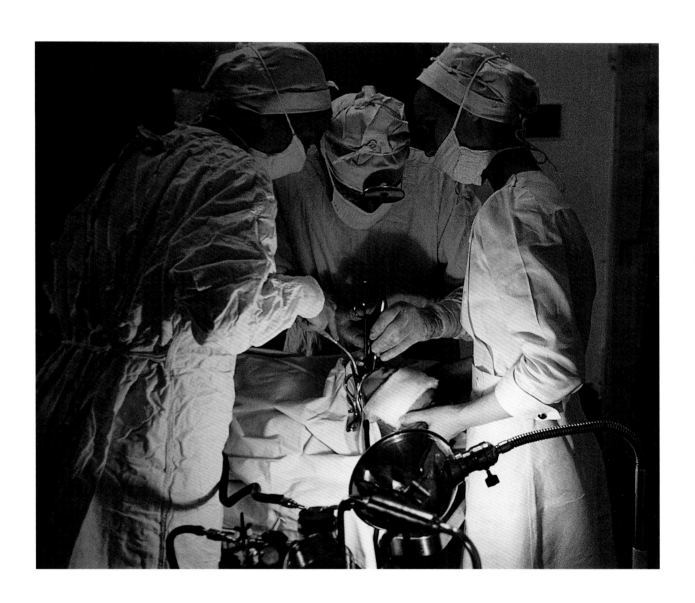

24
Wounded Marine in Oxygen Tent on Board Hospital Ship, USS Solace

Off Shore, Iwo Jima
March 1945

The USS Solace (AH-5) was the only hospital ship in the Pacific when World War II started. On December 7, 1941, she was docked at Pearl Harbor just across the bay from battleship row. She received the first casualties of the war within minutes of the attack. To their horror the staff of the Solace had a special front row seat, only a few hundred yards from the carnage. They helplessly watched as the Japanese torpedo bombers dropped down and flew low alongside the Solace knowing a hospital ship would not fire on them.

The attack on Pearl Harbor taught physicians one lesson in treating the war wounded; it was noted that most of the wounded, even those with relatively minor wounds, who should have survived, died when operated upon immediately. The hypothesis was that the men died because they had sustained both mental and physical trauma. In warfare, when an attack is still going on, the added apprehension of the ongoing battle creates a mental state that perpetuates fear and shock. When a person is in a severe accident or sustains an injury in civilian life, once the accident is over, it's over. There is no anxiety that further injury will be inflicted. This episode taught physicians that unless it was an emergency the wounded should be allowed to rest for a day or two before being operated upon. Once this procedure was in place the death rate plummeted.

Hospital ships were a safe haven in the island campaigns of the Pacific. They allowed respite from battle and relative safety. Only one hospital ship disaster occurred in the Pacific. On April 28, 1945 at 8:42 PM, 30 miles southeast of Okinawa a Japanese kamikaze plane hit the USS Comfort (AH-6). Six doctors, six nurses, nine enlisted men and seven patients were killed. While the Solace was joined by several other hospital ships during the war, she had a special place in World War II history as the ship, which participated in most of the major campaigns in the Pacific. She received wounded at the Solomons, Saipan, Iwo Jima, Eniwetk, Palau, Tarawa and Okinawa. The Burns Collection has the original set of 754 photographs taken on the Solace documenting her tour of duty in WW II. This image was taken March 1945 in the postoperative care unit off the shores of Iwo Jima, and depicts a marine with a chest wound in an oxygen tent attended by the head nurse and a corpsman. In the May 1945 issue of the *Woman's Home Companion*, Patricia Loohridge, a journalist who was on the USS Solace during the battle for Iwo Jima, published a story about her experience.

"The ship was quickly surrounded by a swarm of small boats, the first marine to be carried up made our spines tingle. His chest was swathed in stained bandages "he half rose from the stretcher and sang out, "Hey, Bub, look at that!" In the distance we could see figures struggling up Mt. Suribachi and then we saw it, an American flag on the peak, snapping in the wind. "Helped put her there this morning." Less than an hour had elapsed since he was wounded, now he was safe on the Solace. A doctor quickly looked at his shattered chest and ordered him taken to surgery."

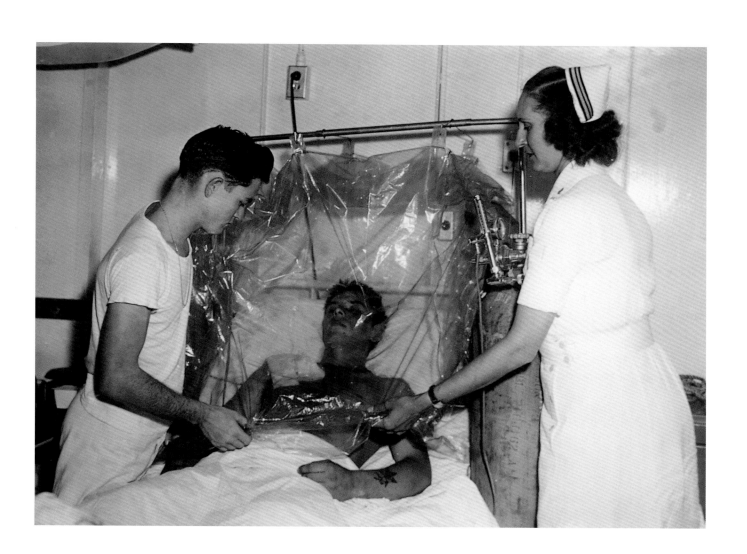

PENICILLIN EXPOSITION:
THE START OF A NEW AGE IN RESPIRATORY AND INFECTIOUS DISEASE THERAPY
PARIS
DECEMBER 1945

This photographic postcard was issued in one of the world's first exhibitions demonstrating the effectiveness and history of penicillin. The most crucial discovery of modern medicine was the creation of the first wonder drug, the antibiotic penicillin. It saved millions of lives, changed the course of history, revolutionized medicine and opened up new fields of research. Respiratory tract disease treatment was dramatically affected. Centuries old scourges, pneumonia, otitis media, pharyngitis, tonsillitis, scarlet fever, diphtheria, and all other primary and secondary infections were forever altered. Penicillin caused an intellectual revolution in society, which now demanded that medical scientists find additional magic bullets that specifically cured a disease.

The discovery of the usefulness of penicillin is surrounded by several myths. Heritage, not actual history, usually is created when important discoveries are made, as those involved make the story seem like a natural progression. It couldn't be further from the truth in the case of penicillin. There were no logical connections between events in the presentation of penicillin. Sir Alexander Fleming (1881-1955) worked at Sir Almoth Wright's Innoculation Department at St. Mary's Hospital in London. In 1928, he discovered that a mold of penicillium inhibited growth of certain bacteria. He reported his findings in 1929 in the *British Journal of Experimental Pathology*. Fleming misinterpreted and misunderstood the phenomena he reported. Physician reaction to his research findings was also unenthusiastic. Fleming focused his career on the concept of a 'Lysozime' surprisingly even after penicillin was recognized as a wonder drug. He was notorious as an ineffective, poor communicator. One associate noted "He had an almost pathologic inability to communicate." In 1939 and 1940, at Oxford University's Sir William Dunn School of Pathology, Ernst Boris Chain, M.D. with Howard W. Flory (1898-1968) developed penicillin into a usable drug. In 1940, Chain et al published in *Lancet*, "Penicillin as a chemotherapeutic agent." These scientists were the brains and promoters of the drug. They demonstrated penicillin was a useful clinical drug that could cure infection 'beyond the wildest dreams of man'; isolated and purified the drug; carried out successful clinical trials; and found out how to produce the drug on a large commercial scale. As England was involved in World War II, the drug was recognized as a powerful secret tool and was immediately subject to secrecy acts. However, the information was shared with the United States Government because they were better able to manufacture the drug in facilities far removed from the war. More importantly the Americans developed a better manufacturing method, a deep fermenting process. Tons of penicillin were produced and shipped to war theaters. In the first six months of 1943 America produced 800 million units and by 1945, 6800 billion units were being produced a year. Penicillin was the Allies' secret weapon. The idea of war is not so much as to kill the enemy but severely wound him. A wounded man takes additional personnel to take care of him. Penicillin allowed the Allies to not only save lives but to send more servicemen back to the front lines. It's curious that Ernst Chain was a German Jew, trained as a physician and bio-chemist and forced to flee Nazi Germany. With his bushy hair he looked much like Einstein and the British offered the genius a post at Oxford. He was very gratified that his discovery made a difference in the war against Germany.

Prior to penicillin, the therapeutic potential of an antibacterial agent was brought to the publics awareness by the development of an effective sulfa drug. Prontisil, the first successful potent drug containing sulphanilamide, was introduced by Gerhard Domagk (1895-1964), Director of Research at Germany's Bayer Company. In 1939, he was awarded the Nobel Prize in Medicine. Another antibiotic, gramicidin, was isolated in 1939 by Rene Jules Dubos. In 1945, Chain, Floury and Fleming shared the Nobel Prize in Medicine.

The years after war became an exciting time in pharmaceutical research as the race to develop new antibiotics started. Few eras have produced as many useful medications. In 1944, Albert Schatz introduced streptomycin; in 1945, Balbina Johnson isolated bacitracin; in 1947, Geoffrey Ainsworth discovered aerosporin (polymixin), John Ehrlich developed chloromycetin and Wallace Herrel produced penicillin G, which substantially prolonged the action of penicillin; in 1948, Benjamin Duggar discovered aureomycin; in 1949, Selman Waxman et al isolated neomycin; in 1950, Alexander Finlay isolated terramycin (oxytetracycline); and in 1951, viomycin and nystatin were isolated. By the end of the century new antibiotic wonder drugs were an expected commodity.

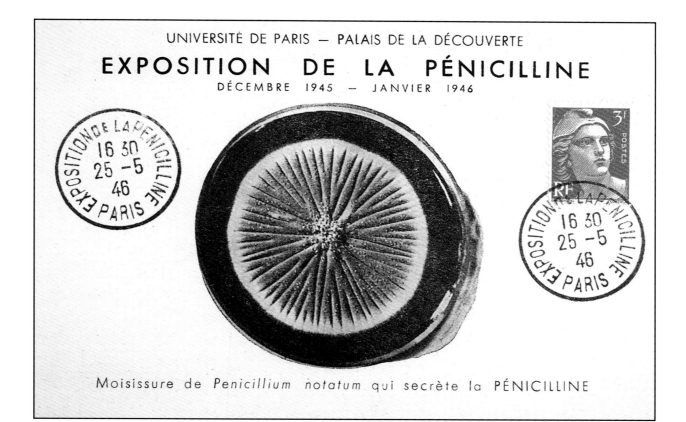

UNIVERSITÉ DE PARIS — PALAIS DE LA DÉCOUVERTE

EXPOSITION DE LA PÉNICILLINE
DÉCEMBRE 1945 — JANVIER 1946

Moisissure de *Penicillium notatum* qui secrète la PÉNICILLINE

BIBLIOGRAPHY

Beck, Emil G., M.D., *Bismuth Paste Injections, Part First, Part Second, Stereo-Clinic*. Southworth Co.: Troy, NY, 1911.

Bernheim, Bertram M., M.D., *The Story of Johns Hopkins: Four Great Doctors and the Medical School they Created*. McGraw Hill Book Co.: New York, NY, 1948.

Bordley III, James, M.D., and A. Harvey McGehee, M.D. *Two Centuries of American Medicine: 1776-1976*. W.B. Saunders Co.: Philadelphia, Pennsylvania, 1976.

Burdick, Gordon G., *X-Ray and High Frequency in Medicine. Physical Therapy.* Library Publishing Co.: Chicago, IL,1909.

Burns, Stanley B., M.D., and Richard Glenner, D.D.S. et al. *The American Dentist: A Pictorial History with a Presentation of Early Dental Photography in America*. Pictorial Histories Publishing Co.: Missoula, MT, 1990.

Burns, Stanley B., M.D., and Ira M. Rutkow, M.D. *American Surgery: An Illustrated History*. Lippincott-Raven Publishers: Philadelphia, PA, 1998.

Burns, Stanley B., M.D. *Early Medical Photography in America: 1839-1883*. The Burns Archive: New York, NY, 1983.

Burns, Stanley B., M.D., and Sherwin Nuland, M.D. et al. *The Face of Mercy: A Photographic History of Medicine at War*. Random House: New York, NY, 1993.

Burns, Stanley B., M.D., and Joel-Peter Witkin, et al. *Masterpieces of Medical Photography: Selections From The Burns Archive*. Twelvetrees Press: Pasadena, CA 1987.

Burns, Stanley B., M.D. *A Morning's Work: Medical Photographs from The Burns Archive & Collection 1843-1939*. Twin Palms Publishers: Santa Fe, New Mexico, 1998.

Burns, Stanley B., M.D., and Jacques Gasser, M.D. *Photographie et Médecine 1840-1880*. Insitut universitaire d'histoire de la santé publique: Lausanne, Switzerland, 1991.

Burns, Stanley B., M.D., and Elizabeth A. Burns. *Sleeping Beauty II: Grief, Bereavement and The Family in Medical Photography, American & European Traditions*. Burns Archive Press: New York, NY, 2002.

Clarke, Edward H., M.D. et al. *A Century of American Medicine: 1776-1876*. Burt Franklin: New York, NY, 1876.

Crowe, Samuel James, M.D., *Halstead of Johns Hopkins: The Man and His Men*. Charles C. Thomas, Publisher: Springfield, Il, 1957.

Cummins, S. Lyle, M.D. *Tuberculosis in History: From the 17th Century to our Times*. Bailliere, Tindall and Cox: London, 1949.

Daniel, Thomas M. and Frederick C. Robbins, Editors. *Polio*. University of Rochester Press: New York, 1997.

Davis, Loyal. *Fifty Years of Surgical Progress: 1905-1955*. Franklin H. Martin Memorial Foundation: Chicago, Illinois, 1955.

Dieffenbach, William H. *Hydrotherapy: A Brief Therapy of the Practical Value of Water in Disease for Students and Practicians of Medicine*. Rebman Co.: New York, NY, 1909.

Donahue, M. Patricia. *Nursing: The Finest Art*. Mosby: St. Louis, Missouri, 1996.

Duffy, John. *The Healers: A History of American Medicine*. University of Illinois Press: Urbana, Illinois, 1976.

Dubos, Rene and Jean. *The White Plague: Tuberculosis, Man and Society*. Little Brown and Company: Boston, MA, 1952.

Dunham, Kennon. *Stereoroentgenography Pulmonary Tuberculosis, Part First and Part Second, Stereo-Clinic*. Southworth Co.: Troy, NY, 1915.

Editors. *Who's Important in Medicine*. Institute for Research in Biography Inc.: New York, NY, 1945.

Fee, Elizabeth and Daniel M. Fox. *AIDS: The Burdens of History*. University of California Press: Berkeley, California, 1988.

Frizot, Michel. *The New History of Photograph.*, Könemann Verlagsgesellschaft mbH: Koln, Germany, 1998.

Fye, W. Bruce, M.D. *The Development of American Physiology: Scientific Medicine in the Nineteenth Century*. Johns Hopkins University Press: Baltimore, Maryland, 1987.

Garrison, Fielding H. M.D. *An Introduction to the History of Medicine. With Medical Chronology, Suggestions for Study and Bibliographic Data*. W.B. Saunders Co.: Philadelphia, Pennsylvania, 1913.

Glaser, Gabrielle. *Doctors Rethinking Treatments for Sick Sinuses*. The New York Times, Health & Fitness Section, Dec. 17, 2002, p. F6.

Gould, Tony. *A Summer Plague: Polio ad Its Survivors*. Yale University Press: New Haven and London, 1995.

Hendrickson, Robert. *More Cunning than Man: A Social History of Rats and Man*. Dorset Press: New York, NY, 1983.

Hersh, Seymour M. *Chemical and Biological Warfare: America's Hidden Arsenal*. Bobbs-Merrill Company: Indianapolis, 1968.

Hochberg, Lew, M.D. *Thoracic Surgery Before the 20th Century.* Vantage Press: New York, NY, 1960.

Hopkins, Donald R. *Princes and Peasants: Smallpox in History*. University of Chicago Press: Chicago and London, 1983.

Hurwitz, Alfred, M.D. and George Degenshein, M.D. *Milestones in Modern Surgery*. Hoeber-Harper, New York, NY, 1958.

Isselbacher, Kurt, M.D., et. al. Eds. *Harrison's Principles of Internal Medicine, Thirteenth Edition*. McGraw Hill: Health Professionals Division, 1994.

Johnson, Stephen L. *The History of Cardiac Surgery: 1896-1955*. Johns Hopkins Press: Baltimore, Maryland, 1970.

Keen, William W. M.D. *Surgery; Its Principles and Practice, by Various Authors*. W.B. Saunders Co.: Philadelphia, PA, 1908.

Kelly, Howard and Walter Burrage. *Dictionary of American Medical Biography*. D. Appleton and Co.: New York, NY, 1928.

Kevles, Bettyann Holtzmann. *Naked to the Bone: Medical Imaging in the Twentieth Century*. Helix Books, Addison Wesley: Reading, Massachusetts, 1997.

Kiple, Kenneth F. *The Cambridge World History of Human Disease*. Cambridge University Press: New York, NY, 1993.

Kovacs, Richard, M.D., *Electrotherapy and Light Therapy: With Essentials of Hydrotherapy and Mechanotherapy*. Lea & Febiger: Philadelphia, 1942.

Leibowitz, J.O. *The History of Coronary Heart Disease*. Wellcome Institute of the History of Medicine: London, 1970.

Levinson, Abraham, M.D. *Pioneers of Pediatrics*. Froben Press: New York, NY, 1936.

Lopate, Carol. *Women in Medicine*. Johns Hopkins Press: Baltimore, Maryland, 1968.

Lyons, Albert S., M.D. and J.S. Petrucelli II, M.D. *Medicine: An Illustrated History*. Harry N. Abrams, Inc.: New York, 1978.

Margotta, Roberto. *The Story of Medicine*. Golden Press: New York, NY, 1967.

Massman, Emory A. *Hospital Ships of World War II: An*

BIBLIOGRAPHY

Illustrated Reference to 39 United States Vessels. McFarland & Co.: Jefferson, NC, 1999.

McHenry, Lawrence C. Jr., M.D. *Garrison's History of Neurology.* Charles C. Thomas: Springfield, IL, 1969.

McNeil, Donald G. *Combined Vaccine Gets F.D.A. Approval,* The New York Times, Dec. 17, 2002, p. A 33.

Morton, Leslie T. *A Medical Bibliography (Garrison and Morton): An Annotated Check-List of Texts Illustrating the History of Medicine.* Andre Deutsch, Morrison & Gibb, Ltd: London, 1970.

Packard, Francis R., M.D. *History of Medicine in the United States.* Hafner Press: New York, NY, 1973.

Parascandola, John, ed. *The History of Antibiotics: A Symposium.* American Institute of the History of Pharmacy: Madison, Wisconsin, 1980.

Puderbach P. *The Massage Operator.* Benedict Lust: Butler, New Jersey, 1925.

Reverby, Susan M. *Ordered to Care: The Dilemma of American Nurisng, 1850-1945.* Cambridge University Press, New York, NY, 1987.

Rice, Thurman B. M.D. *The Conquest of Disease.* Macmillian Co.: New York, NY, 1932.

Rothstein, William G. *American Physicians in the Nineteenth Century: From Sects to Science.* Johns Hopkins University Press: Baltimore, Maryland, 1972.

Rowntree, Leonard G. M.D. *Amid Masters of Twenthieth Century Medicine: A Panorama of Persons and Pictures.* Charles C. Thomas: Springfield, IL, 1958.

Rubin, William, et. al. *Les Demoiselles d'Avignon, tyudies in Modern Art 3, Museum of Modern Art.* Harry Abrams, Inc. Distributors: New York, NY, 1984.

Sarnecky, Mary T. DNSc. *A History of the US Army Nurse Corps.* University of Pennsylvania Press: Philadelphia, PA, 1999.

Schmidt, J.E., M.D. *Medical Discoveries: Who and When.* Charles C. Thomas: Springfield, IL, 1959.

Silverstein, Arthur M. *A History of Immunity.* Academic Press,Inc.: San Diego, 1989.

Tauber, Alfred and Chernyak. *Metchnikoff and the Origins of Immunology: From Metaphor to Theory.* Oxford University Press: New York, NY, 1991

Walker, Kenneth. *The Story of Medicine.* Oxford University Press: New York, 1955.

Wallace, Antony F. *The Progress of Plastic Surgery: An Introductory History.* Willem A. Meeuws: Oxford, England, 1982.

Wangensteen, Owen H., M.D., PhD. and Sarah D. Wangensteen. *The Rise of Surgery: From Empiric Craft to Scientific Discipline.* University of Minnesota Press: Minneapolis, MN, 1978.

Weir, Neil. *Otolaryngology: An Illustrated History.* Butterworths: London, England, 1990.

Wilson, David. *In Search of Penicillin.* Alfred A. Knopf: New York, 1976.

Winslow, Charles-Edward Amory. *The Conquest of Epidemic Disease: A Chapter in the History of Ideas.* University of Wisconsin Press: Madison, WI, 1943.

Worden, Gretchen. *Mütter Museum of the College of Physicians of Philadelphia.* Blast Books: New York, NY, 2002.

Wright, Jonathan, M.D., *A History of Laryngology and Rhinology.* Lea & Febiger: Philadelphia, PA, 1914.

PHOTOGRAPHIC FORMATS

The Evolution of Popular Photographic Processes 1850-1920

In 1851 the wet plate process became the dominant paper photographic process. This method used collodion as a base to hold the silver sensitive material. The solution was then spread over a glass plate. The plate was inserted into the camera, while still wet, exposed while wet, and then immediately developed while still wet. The photographer had to be both a plate maker and processor. Professional photographers produced almost all of the photographs in the 1851-1881 era.

In 1871, a physician, Richard Leach Maddox (1816-1902), changed the nature of photography with his discovery of the dry plate photographic process. A well-known British photomicrographer, Dr. Maddox contributed his images to books on microscopy. He discovered the long searched-for vehicle that had eluded thousands of researchers by using a gelatin bromide base as the sensitive medium instead of collodion. When this gelatin based silver solution dried it could be used at anytime. By 1878 the process was perfected to the degree that it was possible to take photographs in 1/25th of a second.

The dry plate freed the photographer from plate making and gave him greater mobility, as he didn't have to take the developing tanks and apparatus along. If he wished he could simply send the plates to one of the major photographic supply houses for developing and printing. The dry plate allowed thousands of amateurs to join the photographic ranks. In the mid 1880s we begin to see physicians taking private photographs with more intimate poses.

From 1889 forward, anyone could become a photographer. George Eastman introduced to the public a preloaded camera with flexible film capable of 100 photographs. The photographer shot the roll of film and sent the entire camera and film back to Kodak. The photographs were developed and printed, the camera was loaded with another 100 shots and everything was returned to the customer. By 1900, a simpler camera model was introduced named the 'Brownie.' Kodak used the motto "You Press the Button we do the Rest." Physicians could now easily take their own images of patients or their work places. These medical snapshots allowed personal images of the profession. In 1912, Kodak introduced the modern flat flexible 'film' in place of the glass dry plate. It was convenient, thin, lightweight, and unbreakable. It had an important impact in medicine as x-rays could now to be produced with faster exposures times and larger sizes. The 14 by 17 inch chest film became standard.

During the years 1908-1920 the photographic postcard became the most popular size used by the amateur photographer. Billions of these images were produced and sent through the mails. Many of the 'postcards' reproduced in this book are unique, personal images. While we think of the postcard as a commercial production, in this early era both amateur and professional photographers produced them.

The medical photographs in this volume are all originally paper based silver prints or photogravures from silver prints. Because of the relative uniformity of the photographic process the exact type of print has not been identified on each individual photograph in order to concentrate on the subject matter.

DEDICATION

Many physicians who treated and investigated tuberculosis contracted and succumbed to the disease. The list is voluminous and contains many medical luminaries including Dr. Rene Laënnec, inventor of the stethoscope. The sacrifices made by physicians for the advancement of medicine are legendary. Those who died or were mutilated in the development of radiology are well known but the specialists and conquerors fighting tuberculosis have never been fully appreciated. To these selfless individuals, I dedicate this work.

ACKNOWLEDGEMENTS

First and foremost I would like to thank my family who are integral parts of the Burns Archive. They have assisted me, tirelessly, in preparing this historic compilation. My wife, Sara, helps with collecting, cataloging and archiving the collection, and directs the stock photography use of the material. More importantly she serves as my sounding board and editor helping to clarify my ideas. My daughter, Elizabeth, designed and directed the entire production of these volumes from their conception to the final product.

I am most grateful to Saul G. Hornik, MS, RPh, medical marketing consultant. It was his enthusiasm and recognition of the educational importance of my medical, photographic collection, together with his tireless work that made this publication a reality. I give my thanks to Eric Malter, President of MD Communications, for his support of this project. I also wish to express my sincere appreciation to Christopher J. Carney, Director of Training Services of GlaxoSmithKline for understanding the educational value in using the visual history of the past as a foundation for the future.

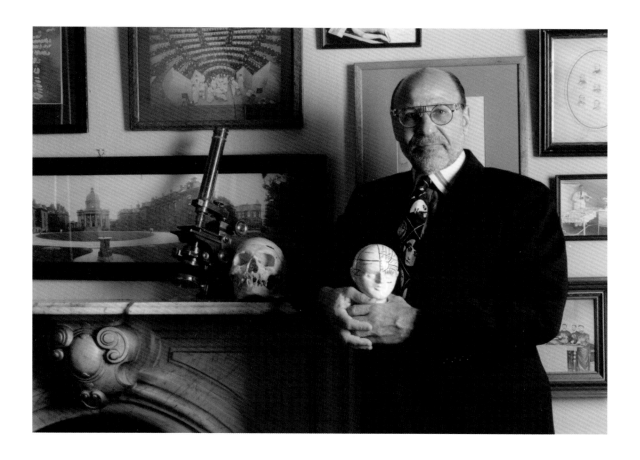

STANLEY B. BURNS, M.D., F.A.C.S.

Stanley B. Burns, M.D., F.A.C.S., a practicing New York City ophthalmic surgeon, is also an internationally distinguished photographic historian, author, curator and collector. His collection, started in 1975, is considered to be the most comprehensive private, early, historic photograph collection in the world. Contained within this archive of over 700,000 vintage prints is the finest and most comprehensive compilation of early medical photographs consisting of 50,000 images taken between 1840 and 1940. These medical photographs have been showcased in countless publications and films, museum exhibitions. France's Channel Plus prepared a documentary on his work as part of the *Great Collectors of the World Series*. Dr. Burns has been an active medical historian since 1970. From 1979-81, he was President of the Medical Archivist of New York State. He has been a member of the medical history departments of The Albert Einstein College of Medicine and The State University of New York, Medical College at Stony Brook; Curator of photographic archives at both The Israeli Institute on The History of Medicine (1978-1993) and The Museum of The Foundation of The American Academy of Ophthalmology. Currently, he is a contributing editor for five specialty medical journals. The Burns Archive, his stock photography and publishing entity, is a valuable photographic resource for both researchers and the media. Using his unique collection Dr. Burns has written ten award-winning photo-history books, hundreds of articles and curated dozens of exhibitions. His film company, Black Mirror Films, produced *Death in America*, a documentary on the history of death practices in America. He is currently working on several medical exhibitions and books, as well as photographic history books on criminology, Judaica, Germans in WW II and African Americans. He can be reached through his web site www.burnsarchive.com.

OTHER BOOKS

Sleeping Beauty II: Grief, Bereavement and The Family in Memorial Photography, American & European Traditions

A Mornings Work: Medical Photographs from The Burns Archive & Collection, 1843-1939

Forgotten Marriage: The Painted Tintype & The Decorative Frame 1860-1910, A Lost Chapter in American Portraiture

American Surgery: An Illustrated History
co-author: Ira M. Rutkow, M.D.

Harm's Way: Lust & Madness, Murder & Mayhem
co-authors: Joel-Peter Witkin, et al

The Face of Mercy: A Photographic History of Medicine at War
co-authors: Matthew Naythons, M.D. and Sherwin Nuland, M.D.

Photographie et Médecine 1840-1880
co-author: Jacques Gasser, M.D.

Sleeping Beauty: Memorial Photography in America

The American Dentist: A Pictorial History
co-authors: Richard Glenner, D.D.S. and Audrey Davis, PhD.

Masterpieces of Medical Photography: Selections From The Burns Archive
co-author: Joel-Peter Witkin

Early Medical Photography in America: 1839-1883

THE BURNS ARCHIVE PRESS
140 EAST 38TH STREET • NEW YORK, N.Y. 10016
TEL: 212-889-1938 • FAX: 212-481-9113 • WWW.BURNSARCHIVE.COM